Cosmetic Industry - Trends, Products and Quality Control

Edited by Selda Pelin Kartal

Published in London, United Kingdom

Cosmetic Industry - Trends, Products and Quality Control
http://dx.doi.org/10.5772/intechopen.1006764
Edited by Selda Pelin Kartal

Contributors
Adina Catinca Grădinaru, Banathi Sihonqo, Bianca Ivănescu, Celenkosini Thembelenkosini Nxumalo, Cristina Lungu, Dongcui Li, Emine Tugba Alatas, Felicia Andrei, Francesco Castellaneta, Gökçe Işıl Kurmuş, Jianhua Zhang, Li Ye, Mariagiovanna Lombardi, Metin Picakciefe, Metin Özaslan, Mokgadi Ursula Makgobole, Ncoza Cordelia Dlova, Nomakhosi Mpofana, Peng Shu, Selda Pelin Kartal, Tian Chen, Xiaoqin Wang, Yuchao Tang, Özlem Karadağ Köse

First published in London, United Kingdom, 2025 by IntechOpen
IntechOpen is the global imprint of INTECHOPEN LIMITED, registered in England and Wales, registration number: 11086078, 167-169 Great Portland Street, London, W1W 5PF, United Kingdom

For EU product safety concerns: IN TECH d.o.o., Prolaz Marije Krucifikse Kozulić 3, 51000 Rijeka, Croatia, info@intechopen.com or visit our website at intechopen.com.

British Library Cataloguing-in-Publication Data
A catalogue record for this book is available from the British Library

Cosmetic Industry - Trends, Products and Quality Control
Edited by Selda Pelin Kartal
p. cm.
Print ISBN 978-1-83634-776-7
Online ISBN 978-1-83634-775-0
eBook (PDF) ISBN 978-1-83634-777-4

If disposing of this product, please recycle the paper responsibly.

Meet the editor

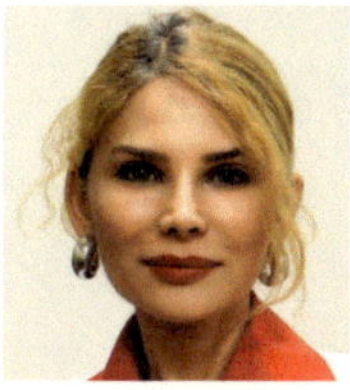

Prof. Dr. Selda Pelin Kartal graduated from Hacettepe University School of Medicine. Currently, she is a Professor and the Head of the Department of Dermatology at the University of Health Sciences, Ministry of Health, Etlik City Hospital in Ankara, Turkey. She has co-authored over 200 published articles and supervised several master's and postdoctoral students. Her actual interests are focused on acne, psoriasis, urticaria, autoimmune bullous diseases, Behçet's disease and cosmetic dermatology.

Contents

Preface

This book aims to provide readers with a comprehensive review of cosmetic applications, the industry, products, trends, and quality control. It is created by experts in various fields and is intended to extend the knowledge about cosmetics, cosmetic procedures, and the industry. I'm grateful to all the contributors and leading experts for submitting their excellent work, which provides an in-depth view of all aspects of the content, backed by the most current literature in the field. I want to extend special thanks to Publishing Process Manager Nina Miocevic for bringing the book to its current form and to my son Demir Durmazlar and Ares for their understanding of the missed family time.

Dr. Selda Pelin Kartal
Professor,
Department of Dermatology and Venereology,
Ministry of Health Etlik City Hospital,
University of Health Science,
Ankara, Turkey

Chapter 1

Aging, Aging Skin, and Anti-Aging Approaches

Emine Tugba Alatas and Metin Picakciefe

Abstract

The number of people aged 60 and over is increasing. This situation will increase even more in the coming years, especially in low- and middle-income countries (LMICs). Aging refers to changes that occur in a person over time and can include psychological, social, physiological, and dermatological changes. Aging of the skin is the decrease in dermatological functions with structural and molecular changes. As we know, UV has a very important role in vitamin D synthesis. However, unprotected exposure to UV rays can cause skin aging. In this review, aging, skin aging, anti-aging approaches, the effects of solar radiation, and antioxidants on aging were examined from the perspective of dermatology.

Keywords: aging, aging skin, anti-aging approaches, sun, protection

1. Introduction

Everyone should have the opportunity to live a long and healthy life all over the world. However, our environment can be beneficial to both physical and mental health, as well as harmful. The environment plays a huge role in our behavior and exposure to health risks (e.g., air pollution), our access to services (e.g., health and social care), and the shortcomings of aging. The number and proportion of people aged 60 and over in the population are increasing. The number of people aged 60 and over was 1 billion in 2019. This number is expected to increase to 1.4 billion in 2030 and 2.1 billion in 2050. The increase in the elderly population is taking place at a rapid pace and will accelerate in the coming years, especially in low- and middle-income countries (LMICs) [1].

Technological and medical advances in the last century have significantly extended the lifespan of people. Average life expectancy in developed countries has increased by nearly 20 years since 1950, and it is estimated that almost 10% of people living in developed countries will be 80 years or older by 2050 [2, 3]. However, there is a significant gap in their overall healthy living, meaning that people may experience functional limitations [4]. Adding to the increasing health costs, it leads to an increasing burden on society. Low physical activity and high sedentary time can be seen due to biological aging mechanisms and lifestyle behaviors [3].

Biological aging rates vary widely among individuals [5]. Aging age is defined as the biological and physiological reserve of an individual at a given time [6].

Therefore, measuring biological aging informs the need for lifestyle interventions before aging becomes an adverse clinical event and is a crucial challenge with significant public health implications [7].

In this review, aging, skin aging, anti-aging strategies, the effects of solar radiation, and antioxidants on aging are mentioned.

2. Aging

Aging causes changes and opportunities in the person. Demand for primary health care and long-term care will increase, resulting in a larger and better-trained workforce and more age-friendly physical and social environments. Still, these investments can bring many benefits to older people, whether within the family or within the local community (e.g., on a voluntary basis or in the formal or informal workforce). Societies that adapt to these changing demographics and invest in healthy aging can enable individuals to live longer and healthier lives [1].

Healthy aging is known as the development and maintenance of the ability that provides well-being in older ages. Functional ability is constituted by the individual's internal capacity (i.e., the individual's physical and mental capacities), the environment in which he lives (including, in the broadest sense, the physical, social, and political environments), and the interactions between them [1].

3. Skin aging

Skin Aging is a dynamic and multifactorial process and occurs in two different ways. Natural (intrinsic) aging is an inevitable condition that develops depending on genetic structure and time. Telomeres, located at the ends of chromosomes, are thought to play a role at the cellular level [8]. Natural and progressive telomere shortening is one of the primary mechanisms of cellular aging in the skin. Telomeres and other cell structures are also affected by oxidative damage resulting from cellular metabolism [9].

Extrinsic (extrinsic) changes in aging are usually preventable and result from external factors such as smoking, malnutrition, and sun exposure. Among the external factors, exposure to the sun is reported to be the cause of 80% of the aging seen in the skin, especially in the facial skin [10].

4. Changes in the skin as a result of aging

The changes that occur with aging are seen in the epidermis, dermis, and subcutaneous tissue. The changes seen in the epidermis layer with aging have been revealed by a number of studies. Although it is accepted that the epidermis becomes thinner due to aging, El-Domyati et al. reported that the epidermal thickness of the skin exposed to the sun was greater in their study comparing sun-exposed and sun-protected skin samples [11]. Another study showed that the spinal layer within the wrinkles is thinner than the adjacent tissue [12]. The most striking change is the flattening of the dermoepidermal junction. The indentation of the dermoepidermal junction protects the skin from mechanical effects. The area between these two surfaces decreases as a result of the erasure of dermal papillae and epidermal rete lines with aging. This leads to the weakening of communication between the two parts, a reduction in skin fragility, and damage to the nutrient transfer between the dermis and epidermis [13].

In aged skin, melanocytes are larger and morphologically more heterogeneous. The decrease in the number of melanocytes with age and the deterioration of pigment transfer to keratinocytes cause irregular pigmentation and a decrease in the protective barrier against UV rays.

The most striking changes related to aging in the dermis are seen in collagen, elastin, and glycosaminoglycans. In aged skin, collagen fibrils are thickened and arranged in rope-like bundles. While 80% type I and 15% type III collagen are found in young skin, type I collagen decreases with age [14]. Type I collagen is also reduced in UV-exposed skin [14, 15]. The degree of this reduction is proportional to the severity of the photodamage. Type IV collagen is the main collagen in the dermoepidermal junction and is of great importance for mechanical interaction. With aging, deregulation of collagen fibers in the dermis and abnormal accumulation of elastin-containing substances are observed [16].

Age-related clinical and histological changes in the skin due to the sun are more dramatic and different than those of sun-protected skin. Usually, the problems occur in open areas such as the face, chest, and outer surfaces of the arms.

5. Theories of aging

1. Cell cycle theory
2. Oxidation-reduction theory
3. Mutation theory
4. Free radical theory
5. Immunological theory

5.1 Cell cycle theory

Human and animal cells have a limited division capacity, which has been demonstrated in vivo and in vitro. As age progresses, DNA damage increases, repair decreases, and the number of cells and their capacity to divide decrease, as a result of which the regeneration ability of the tissues weakens and atrophy is observed. In each cell cycle, telomeres (terminal parts of eukaryotic chromosomes) shorten in length, and when this decrease reaches a certain level, the cell cycle pauses and apoptosis develops. Replication of telomeres is only possible in early young cells. The positive and negative effects of some other proteins on the genes controlling cell division (on the 1, 4th, and 7th chromosomes) may also be decisive [17].

5.2 Oxidation-reduction theory

This theory considers life as a chain of reactions, and it is accepted that life expectancy and rate of aging depend on the amount of reactants and the rate of reaction. The completion of the reaction sequences is the end of life. With the genetically determined metabolic potential, the metabolic rate determines the length of life and the rate of aging. Environmental factors can also affect this speed. If we make a more understandable interpretation of this assumption, it can be evaluated as "aging battery weakens, death is battery depletion". Unfortunately, these batteries are disposable and not "Rechargeable" [17].

5.3 Mutation theory (nucleic acid degradation)

In this theory, disruption of homeostasis in the cell is attributed to the disorder in nucleic acid functions. Disturbances in nucleic acid structure and functions, which may occur due to various reasons, are thought to be an important cause of aging. In another theory, it is thought that the disruption of the control of prevention, detection, repair, and replacement in the damage control system of mutations in genes is effective. There may be deterioration in the structures of DNAs, mRNA synthesis may be inhibited, or faulty mRNAs may occur (Mutations may occur spontaneously or under the influence of free radicals and UV). These mutations lead to the loss of genetic control, and in such cases, even a small loss can be highly detrimental, as most of the energy is spent repairing these disorders. At this point, the assumption intersects with the previous finite energy assumption [17].

5.4 Free radical theory

It is an opinion that accepts the fact that free radicals that occur due to various reasons (stress, smoking, UV, air pollution, radiation, destructive drugs, etc.) have a very important role in the aging function, causing damage to many tissues, especially DNA. It is one of the most popular assumptions. Regardless of their origin, free oxygen radicals are one of the important causes that accelerate the aging process by causing cell damage. Free radicals inactivate enzymes, break down DNA by oxidation, and break down unsaturated fats, leading to lipid peroxidation, destruction, and carcinogenesis also begin. Oxidative damage also affects telomeres and accelerates telomere shortening. The destruction of connective tissue and cellular matrix plays a very important role in the aging process. Free radicals contribute to the aging process by inhibiting the TGF-Beta effect and collagen I and III synthesis. While collagen decreases, degradation enzymes such as collagenase, gelatinase, and stromelysin-1 increase. In addition, the DNA of mitochondria, which are the organelles that produce energy, is also destroyed, leading to reduced function and affecting energy production.

These decrease with age, and as a result, it is thought that destruction may increase, leading to deterioration of chromatin configuration, which may lead to loss of genetic control [17].

5.5 Immunological theory

With age, the functions of antigen-presenting cells, antigen-specific B and T cells, and lymphocyte cytokine secretions decrease. The levels of pro-inflammatory cytokines and oxidative stress increase. As a result of the loss of the self-recognition feature of the organism, autoimmune reactions may develop and cause destruction in cells and systems. Atrophy of the thymus by shrinking with age, cellular differentiation, and regression of other thymic functions can be interpreted as the beginning of this event [17].

5.5.1 Hormones

Hormonal changes experienced in menopause in women and in advanced ages in men also have an important place in aging. Due to the decrease in pituitary, adrenal, and gonadal secretions, circulating hormone levels decrease. The skin, both as a target organ and as an endocrine organ, is greatly affected by these reductions. In women, 17 beta-estradiol, DHEA, DHEA-SO4, GH, and IGF (insulin-like GH) are significantly reduced. Especially, the sudden decrease in estrogen after menopause causes a decrease in skin blood flow and a decrease in the stimulating effect on fibroblasts. As a result, a decrease in collagen amount and hydration, a decrease in mucopolysaccharide and hyaluronic acid synthesis, a change in the ratio of glycosaminoglycans, and thinning of the skin are observed [18].

5.5.2 Smoking

Smokers (more than five years, <a pack of cigarettes a day) have increased lines and wrinkles, facial dryness, atrophy, and a grayish color and a dull, dark orange erythema. Especially, the wrinkles on the lips are characteristic. In the longer term, a yellowish, coarsened skin appears. These findings are added to the others and are potentiated by sun exposure. In addition, it has been reported that the constricting effect of smoking on the vessels may also contribute to the aging process, partially, by creating regional dermal ischemia, with oxygenation and nutrition problems. It is considered to cause elastosis. While some studies have reported that smokers experience skin aging twice as much as non-smokers, some studies have shown that the effect of smoking without sun factor is very low, and it has been claimed that smoking may have a phototoxic effect [17].

5.5.3 Nutrition

Nutritional habits may also affect the skin aging process indirectly, although not directly. Inadequate nutrition, especially as a result of intense diets, may cause an increase in tissue destruction by preventing adequate intake of proteins, vitamins, and minerals necessary for antioxidant struggle in the organism [1].

5.5.4 Dry skin

Although the opinions that dry skin and irritation due to external factors increase skin aging and that dry skin wrinkles more easily come to the fore from time to time, these events are temporary and the skin will return to normal when conditions return to normal. In addition, skin dryness seems to be a consequence of skin aging rather than a cause [1].

5.5.5 Gravity

Apart from these, sagging of the skin is one of the important signs of aging and depends on natural gravity as well as connective tissue degeneration [1].

During the normal aging process of the skin, which is the outermost part of our body, as a result of cell metabolism, reactive oxygen derivatives such as superoxide radicals, hydrogen peroxide, and hydroxyl radicals are produced that can easily react with other molecules. Short-term exposure of key biological molecules such as lipids and proteins with these structures can cause damage [18]. The most basic damage seen in the skin is the formation of structures that cause erythema and inflammation by changing the lipid structure of the skin. These changes cause irreversible defects in the basic elements (elastin and collagen fibers) in the protein and amino acid structure of the skin. Therefore, ROS is today recognized as the most important cause of skin aging [18].

When sunlight combines with the oxygen-rich atmosphere, it causes undesirable and harmful effects on the skin. These effects can be either acute or chronic. Acute effects include erythema, edema, and hyperpigmentation. Chronic effects include photoaging, photocarcinogenicity, and suppression of the immune system. Photoaging causes changes in the skin such as wrinkles, dryness, and variegated pigment anomalies such as hyperpigmentation and hypopigmentation. In the initiation of photochemical reactions in the skin, the UV rays from the sun must be absorbed by the chromophore in order to initiate the photochemical reaction series that results in skin cancer or photoaging [18, 19]. These photochemical reactions cause changes in DNA, including the oxidation of nucleic acids. Oxidative reactions can make modifications that result in changes in the function of proteins and lipids. Their accumulation can also cause aging in tissues. In order to reduce these changes, the human body is equipped with a mechanism that uses natural antioxidant enzymes and non-enzymatic antioxidants to cope with oxidative stress. However, sunlight and other free radical-generating factors (e.g., smoking and air pollution) can upset this system, and insufficient natural protection results in oxidative damage.

Since oral antioxidants cannot reach the skin in effective concentration, topical application is preferred in the treatment of skin aging and photoaging. The purpose of using antioxidants, which serve as cosmeceutical/dermocosmetic raw materials, is to replace the decreased amount of physiological antioxidants that form the natural defense mechanism of the skin [18].

6. Approaches to mitigate skin aging

Skin aging is the deterioration of dermatological functions that develop with structural and molecular changes. Various approaches have been proposed to reverse this situation. These approaches can be summarized as follows:

Preventive measures (sun protection, smoking cessation), Medical treatment (Tretinoin, vitamin C, Vitamin D, Vitamin E Moisturizers, Alpha hydroxy acids), Skin rejuvenation (Chemical peeling, Dermabrasion, Laser ablation), Injection of fillers (Autogenic fillers, Allogeneic fillers, Xerogenic fillers, Synthetic fillers), Botulinum toxin injection, Alpha lipoic acid, Coenzyme Q10 (Ubiquinone), Lycopene, Tea Polyphenols, Silymarin, Coffee Extract, Grape Seed Extract, Pomegranate Extract, Niacinamide, Aloe vera gel [8].

Sunscreens are the gold standard for photoaging protection. Sunscreens can be formulated physically, chemically, or in combination. The effectiveness of a sunscreen product is based on its Sun Protection Factor (SPF). As the SPF value increases, the protection increases. Sunscreens should be applied to the skin areas half an hour before going out in the sun and should be reapplied every two hours if sun exposure continues. In addition to sunscreen, physical coverings such as sunglasses and hats should be used [19, 20].

Antioxidants prevent oxidative stress in body tissues by neutralizing toxic oxygen molecules and free radicals, thereby protecting cell membranes [18]. The most commonly used substances in products for antioxidant purposes consist of molecules such as Vitamins (A, C, E, and B vitamins), Alpha-lipoic acid, Coenzyme Q-10 (ubiquinol), Idebenone, Polyphenols, and Kinetin. The protection of these substances against inflammation, photodamage, and cancer formation is different from each other [18].

6.1 Alpha lipoic acid

Lipoic acid, which is found physiologically in human cells, is the strongest antioxidant substance in the cosmetic market today, which is frequently added to the formulations of anti-aging cosmetic products. It increases cell metabolism in the skin and helps to repair aged skin while preventing future damage. With aging, glutathione levels naturally decrease, making you more susceptible to free radicals and other environmental toxins. ALA restores the level of glutathione, a protective antioxidant, and detoxification compounds to near normal [18].

6.2 Coenzyme Q10 (ubiquinone)

Coenzyme Q10 (CoQ10), or ubiquinone, is a fat-soluble antioxidant found in all human cells as a component of the respiratory chain, as well as in foods such as fish and shellfish. Up to 95% of the body's energy needs are provided by CoQ10. Its powerful antioxidant property comes from its ability to scavenge free oxygen derivatives and protect cells from oxidative stress. It is found in all tissues, especially the skin, and is believed to play a role in both extrinsic and chronological aging processes. It has been reported by many authors that the level of CoQ10 in tissues decreases with age [18].

6.3 Lycopene

Lycopene, a powerful antioxidant, is a carotenoid found in red fruits and vegetables that scavenges the free radicals responsible for their red color. In addition to its protective feature against premature aging, it also provides antioxidant protection against environmental damage. Lycopene strengthens the skin by increasing its ability to produce collagen and reducing wrinkles. It has been proven in mouse models to have chemopreventive effects against photo-induced tumors. Although there is little clinical data on it, it is included in the composition of various skin care products [18].

6.4 Tea polyphenols

Green tea is a very popular beverage and is an antioxidant extracted from the *Camellia sinensis* plant. Green tea mainly contains monomer catechins such as epicatechin, epicatechin-3-gallate, epigallocatechin, and epigallocatechin-3-gallate. Topically applied green tea extracts both help maintain the levels of glutathione and glutathione recycling enzymes in UV-exposed skin and reduce the depletion of skin-protective antioxidant enzymes [18].

6.5 Silymarin

Silymarin is an antioxidant, a natural polyphenolic flavonolignan derived from the seeds of the plant *Silybum marianum* (milk thistle). Silibin (silibinin) is the main component that is considered the most biologically active and has powerful antioxidant properties. Thanks to its antioxidant, anti-inflammatory, and immune-regulating properties, it helps prevent skin cancer and photoaging [18].

6.6 Coffee extract

It is an antioxidant extracted from the fruit of the Coffee arabica plant containing polyphenols and has a stronger antioxidant property than green tea, pomegranate extract, and vitamins C and E [18].

6.7 Grape seed extract

Grape seed extract is extracted from the plant *Vitis vinifera* and contains proanthocyanidins from the flavonoid family. It is a powerful antioxidant with free radical scavenging activity, and this effect is stronger than vitamins C and E. It is added to topical cosmetic formulations as an anti-aging. It is also effective in healing hair care products. Takahashi et al. determined that they increase the division of epithelial cells in hair follicles in mice and it is more effective than minoxidil [18].

6.8 Pomegranate extract

Pomegranate extract can be obtained from various parts of the *Punica granatum* plant. Especially, phenolic components have strong antioxidant activity. Topical application of fruit extract has been shown in vitro to ameliorate UVA and UVB-mediated skin damage [18].

6.9 Niacinamide

Niacinamide, or nicotinamide, is a water-soluble component of the vitamin B complex group. Besides antioxidant activity, it has also been shown to exhibit anti-inflammatory, lightening, and immunomodulatory properties. The use of niacinamide has been shown to improve texture and skin tone and reduce fine lines, wrinkles, and hyperpigmentation [18].

6.10 Aloe vera gel

It is a herbal extract that has been used in cosmetic products for many years and obtained from the leaves of the Aloe vera plant, which has moisturizing and softening effects on the skin. It has an anti-inflammatory effect due to the sterols it carries. It also has a UVA filtering feature due to its cinnamic acid esters. For this reason, it is used to delay the formation of signs of aging against aging caused by UV rays and free radicals [18].

No matter how we define it, aging is an elusive, natural, general, and irreversible, but inevitable physiological event. Skin aging is a process that develops over time and progresses with natural and external effects. In this process, the sun is one of the factors that increase skin aging. Premature skin aging due to sun rays is an issue that concerns the general public. Although there is a certain awareness on this issue, a full level of knowledge on protection has not been reached yet. In this review, skin aging, the effects of solar radiation, and antioxidants on aging are mentioned [18].

Further investigation is still needed to fill the remaining gaps in the literature, especially regarding the hallmarks that suffer from a lack of studies, including genomic instability, telomere attrition, epigenetic changes, and cellular senescence [7].

The historically significant change in the global population requires adaptations to the way societies are structured across all sectors, including health and social care, transportation, housing, and urban planning. Working to make the world more age-friendly is an essential and urgent part of our changing demographics. Societies that adapt to this changing demographic and invest in healthy aging can enable individuals to live both longer and healthier lives and for societies to reap the dividends [1].

Author details

Emine Tugba Alatas[1*] and Metin Picakciefe[2]

1 Department of Dermatology, Mugla Sitki Kocman University, Mugla, Turkey

2 Faculty of Medicine, Department of Public Health, Mugla Sitki Kocman University, Mugla, Turkey

*Address all correspondence to: dretuba_oz@hotmail.com

References

[1] Şen T. Skin aging and importance of antioxidants. Ankara Üniversitesi Eczacılık Fakültesi dergisi / Journal of Faculty of Pharmacy of Ankara University. 2016;**40**:36-53

[2] Utto J. Understanding premature skin aging. The New England Journal of Medicine. 1997;**337**:1463-1465

[3] El-Domyati M, Attia S, Saleh F, Brown D, Birk DE, Gasparro F, et al. Intrinsic aging vs. Photoaging: A comparative histopathological, immunohistochemical, and ultrastructural study of skin. Experimental Dermatology. 2002;**11**:398-405

[4] Contet-Audonneau JL, Jeanmarie C, Pauly GA. Histological study of human wrinkle structures: Comparison between sun-exposed areas of the face, with or without wrinkles, and sun-protected areas. British Journal of Dermatology. 1999;**131**:717-725

[5] Yaar M, Glichrest A. Ageing and photoageing of keratinocytes and melanocytes. Clinical Experimental Dermatology. 2001;**26**:583-591

[6] Gniadecka M, Nielsen OF, Wessel S, Heidenheim M, Christensen DH, Wulf HC. Water and protein structure in photoaged and chronically aged skin. Journal of InvestigativeDermatology. 1998;**111**:1129-1133

[7] Fisher GJ, Wang ZQ, Datta SC, Varani J, Kang S, Voorhees JJ. Pathophysiology of premature skin aging induced by UV light. The New England Journal of Medicine. 1997;**37**:1419-1427

[8] Varani J, Spearman D, Perone P, Fligiel SEG, Datta SC, Wang ZQ, et al. Inhibition of type I procollagen synthesis by damaged collagen in photoaged skin and by collagenase-degraded collagen in vitro. American Journal of Pathology. 2001;**158**:931-942

[9] Ma W, Wlaschek M, Tantcheva-Poor I, Schneider LA, Naderi L, Razi-Wolf Z, et al. Chronological ageing and photoageing of the fibroblasts and the dermal connective tissue. Clinical and Experimental Dermatology. 2001;**6**:592-599

[10] Shyam BV. Dermatology for the elderly: An Indian perspective. Clinics in Dermatology. 2011;**29**:91-96

[11] Palmer SJ. Dermatological conditions in older adults: Clinical overview. British Journal of Community Nursing. 2020;**25**(5):222-226

[12] Aydemir EH. Skin Aging. Okmeydanı Tıp Dergisi. 2013;**29**(Ek sayı 2):89-93

[13] Rinnerthaler M, Bischof J, Streubel MK, Trost A, Richter K. Oxidative stress in aging human skin. Biomolecules. 2015;**5**(2):545-589

[14] Trautinger F. Mechanisms of photodamage of skin and its functional consequences for skin ageing. Clinical and Experimental Dermatology. 2001;**26**:573-577

[15] Amer M, Maged M. Cosmeceuticals versus pharmaceuticals. Clinical Dermatology. 2009;**27**:428-430

[16] Kerscher M, Buntrock H. Update on cosmeceuticals. Journal der Deutschen Dermatologischen Gesellschaft. 2011;**9**:314-328

[17] Stone WL, Smith M. Therapeutic uses of antioxidant liposomes. Molecular Biotechnology. 2004;**27**:217-230

[18] Choi CM, Berson DS. Cosmeceuticals. Seminar in Cutaneous Medicine Surgery. 2006;**25**:163-168

[19] Chen L, Hu JY, Wang SQ. The role of antioxidants in photoprotection: A critical review. Journal of American Academic Dermatology. 2012;**67**:1013-1024

[20] Alatas ET, Kara Polat A, Doğan G, Piçakçiefe M. Assessment of the academic staff's knowledge, attitudes and habits related to sun protection and sunscreen use. Turkish Journal of Dermatology. 2018;**12**:9-17

Chapter 2

Sensory Science in Cosmetics

Felicia Andrei

Abstract

This chapter explores the critical role that sensory science plays in the creation and assessment of cosmetics. It investigates how consumer preferences and product effectiveness are influenced by sensory perception, which includes touch, sight, smell, and even sound. The chapter demonstrates how sensory qualities like texture, scent, and esthetic appeal are carefully designed to improve user happiness and emotional involvement by fusing concepts from psychology, physiology, and material science. It also covers cutting-edge techniques for measuring and improving these qualities, such as sensory panels and instrumental assessments. This thorough analysis highlights how art and science may work together to create cosmetics that appeal to a wide range of consumer wants and sensibilities.

Keywords: cosmetic product development, multisensory experience, visual appeal, emotional engagement, sensory science, texture analysis, consumer preferences

1. Introduction

1.1 Overview of sensory science and its relevance to cosmetics

Sensory science is pivotal in the cosmetics industry by bridging the gap between formulation, consumer satisfaction, and emotional connection to products. Tactile attributes, such as smoothness, spreadability, and absorbency, are critical in defining the feel and usability of products, directly impacting consumer satisfaction and repurchase behavior.

Fragrance, a key component of sensory design, goes beyond mere appeal by evoking emotions, memories, and a sense of identity, often becoming a brand's hallmark. Even auditory cues, such as the click of a well-designed cap or the fizz of an aerosol, contribute subtly to the overall experience, reinforcing perceptions of quality and innovation.

The integration of sensory science into product development allows cosmetic brands to create offerings that align with consumer expectations while standing out in a competitive market. Cultural and demographic differences also influence sensory preferences, prompting brands to tailor formulations and marketing strategies to resonate with diverse audiences globally.

Looking ahead, the future of sensory science in cosmetics will be shaped by personalization and sustainability. Advances in technology enable brands to design products that cater to individual sensory profiles, providing tailored experiences for unique skin types and preferences.

1.2 Literature research

The field was examined in research papers from various websites like: Science Direct, Research Gate, JSTOR, SAGE Journals, Intech Open, Elsevier, EPRA, IJRASET, and so on, offering a thorough overview of the current literature and theoretical frameworks.

I found an increasing number of articles published especially in the last two decades (**Figure 1**), as well as a general interest and many citations since the introduction of the databases (**Figure 2**). A chart of documents published over time on a specific topic provides insights into research trends, historical context, and the impact of scholarly work. It helps identify emerging subtopics, collaborative networks, and shifts in interest.

The main themes identified in the provided abstracts are "sensory evaluation methodologies," "cross-cultural sensory perception," and "the role of rheology in cosmetic formulations." The topic map created shows the relationship between themes, determined by documents covering the same topics (**Figure 3**).

The size of the bubble indicates how many documents are on this topic, while the arrows show which topics reference each other.

The visualization of the fields of publications in the core collections can be seen in the figure below (**Figure 4**).

1.3 Definition of sensory science and its interdisciplinary nature

Sensory science is a multidisciplinary field investigating how humans perceive, interpret, and respond to sensory stimuli through the interaction of sensory organs and the brain. In the context of product development, such as cosmetics, food, and consumer goods, sensory science seeks to evaluate and optimize sensory attributes to enhance usability, satisfaction, and emotional engagement. These include: Psychology, Physiology, Material Science and many more.

Sensory science heavily relies on psychology to explore how sensory stimuli influence human emotions, cognition, and behavior.

- Cognitive psychology investigates how individuals process and interpret sensory information, including the role of memory, attention, and expectations in shaping perception. For instance, in cosmetics, packaging color or branding may create expectations of product quality or effectiveness, which in turn influence perceived performance.

- Behavioral psychology studies consumer reactions to sensory attributes under controlled conditions, helping identify patterns in preferences and

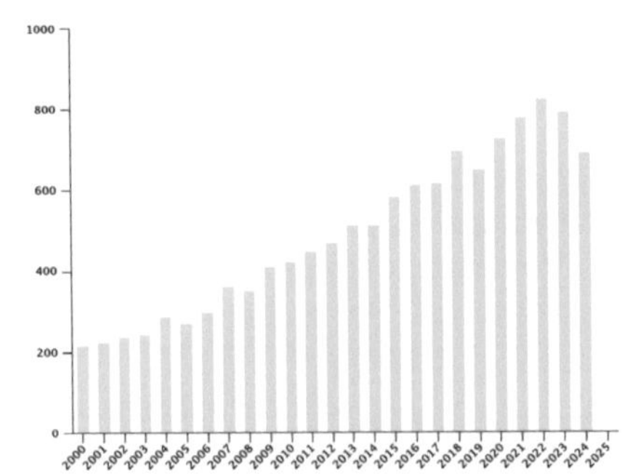

Figure 1.
Documents over time.

DOI: http://dx.doi.org/10.5772/intechopen.1009804

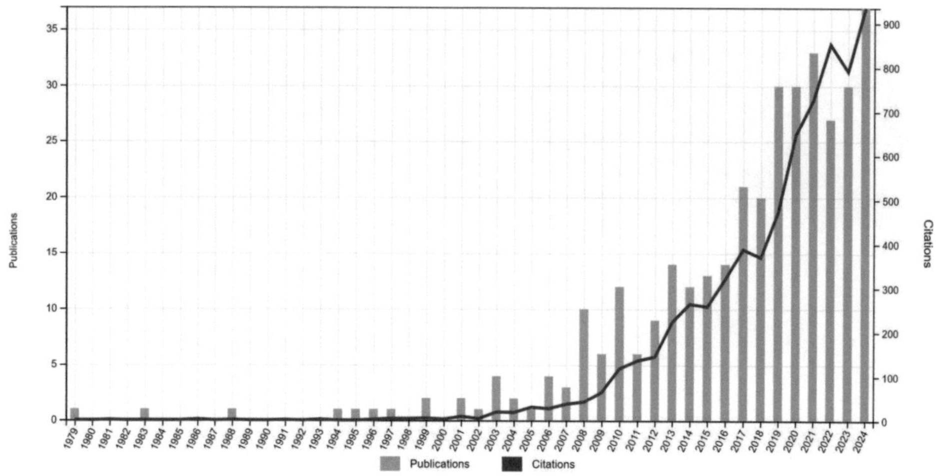

Figure 2.
Publications and citations over time.

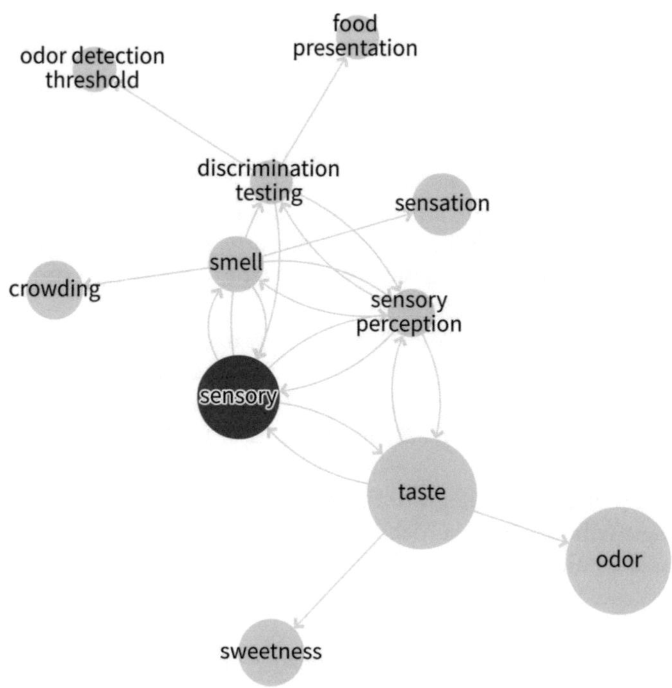

Figure 3.
The topic map.

decision-making. Behavioral insights guide sensory testing, such as blind tests to isolate sensory attributes from brand bias.

- Emotional psychology explores how sensory inputs, such as a soothing texture or pleasant fragrance, evoke emotions like relaxation, happiness, or confidence. Emotional branding leverages this connection to create products that foster loyalty and emotional attachment.

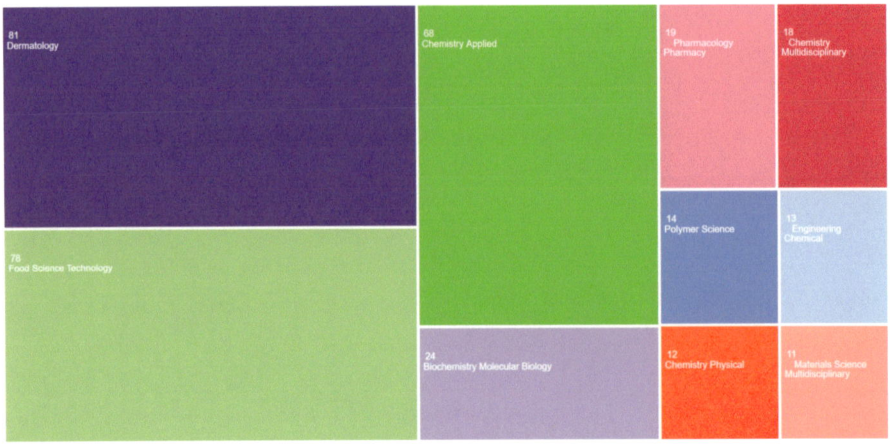
81
Dermatology
68
Chemistry Applied
19
Pharmacology Pharmacy
18
Chemistry Multidisciplinary
78
Food Science Technology
14
Polymer Science
13
Engineering Chemical
24
Biochemistry Molecular Biology
12
Chemistry Physical
11
Materials Science Multidisciplinary

Figure 4.
The visual map of the journals of publication.

Physiology provides the foundation for understanding the biological mechanisms underlying sensory perception. Sensory science studies how receptors or sensory organs in the eyes, skin, nose, tongue, and ears detect stimuli (e.g., light, pressure, chemical compounds) and transmit signals to the brain for interpretation on neural pathways. Understanding these pathways helps in designing products that align with the sensory thresholds and preferences of the target audience. Physiological factors such as age, gender, health conditions, and genetics influence sensory perception. For example, aging skin may perceive textures differently, while genetic differences can affect olfactory sensitivity. This knowledge allows for personalized product development tailored to specific demographics.

In cosmetics, physiological studies focus on how ingredients interact with the skin, influencing sensory attributes like smoothness, spreadability, and absorption [1].

Material science is also critical in creating products with optimal sensory characteristics, such as texture, viscosity, and appearance.

- Texture and rheology: Rheological studies analyze how materials flow and deform, influencing attributes like spreadability, creaminess, and adhesion. Innovations in material science allow formulators to create textures that transform during application, such as gel-to-foam cleansers or lightweight emulsions [2].

- Surface interactions: Material science examines how products interact with surfaces, such as how a cream feels on the skin or how a fragrance diffuses in the air. These interactions determine the sensory experience and influence consumer preferences.

- Sustainability in materials: Recent advancements focus on developing eco-friendly materials that maintain desirable sensory attributes, such as biodegradable textures and natural fragrances. This aligns with growing consumer demand for sustainable and environmentally conscious products.

The interdisciplinary nature of sensory science lies in its ability to combine these diverse fields into a cohesive framework for understanding and optimizing sensory experiences: Psychology helps identify consumer needs, desires, and emotional responses to sensory stimuli. Physiology explains the biological mechanisms of perception and highlights individual differences in sensory thresholds. Material science provides the tools and techniques to design products that deliver desired sensory attributes. By integrating these disciplines, sensory science enables the development of products that go beyond functionality to deliver holistic, multi-sensory experiences [3, 4].

1.4 Historical evolution of sensory evaluation in cosmetic development

The roots of sensory evaluation in cosmetics can be traced back to ancient civilizations, where beauty products were crafted using natural ingredients like oils, clays, and plant extracts. The early beginnings were in the artisanal era, and while there was no structured sensory testing, the importance of sensory attributes was evident in the meticulous preparation of these products, which were often reserved for royalty or the elite.

The nineteenth and early twentieth centuries saw the transformation of cosmetics from handcrafted items to mass-produced goods, driven by advancements in industrial technology. During the Industrial Revolution, standardization and innovation caused the sensory evaluation to become more systematic, as manufacturers sought uniformity and appeal. The sensory characteristics of these innovations, from smoother creams to vibrant lipsticks, became central to product appeal. While consumer feedback was still largely anecdotal, the foundation for modern sensory science was being laid.

After World War II, the cosmetics industry experienced a boom, with brands expanding their offerings to cater to a broader, more diverse audience. Sensory evaluation became a formalized process as companies recognized the importance of understanding consumer preferences. The mid-twentieth century came with the rise of consumer-centric testing, and marketing began emphasizing sensory appeal, using slogans and imagery to evoke emotions tied to the product experience.

By the 1980s and 1990s, sensory evaluation had evolved into a scientific discipline integral to cosmetic research and development. Descriptive sensory analysis, where trained panels systematically quantified specific product attributes, became standard practice. The late twentieth century was the time of the integration of sensory science. Multinational companies invested heavily in sensory science labs to refine their formulations and ensure global appeal across diverse markets.

In the twenty-first century, sensory evaluation has become more sophisticated, reflecting the integration of advanced technologies and changing consumer expectations. Multisensory experiences and personalization, digital tools, artificial intelligence, and big data are now used to predict and optimize sensory profiles, allowing brands to tailor products to individual preferences. Textures that transform upon application (e.g., gel-to-foam cleansers) and products with interactive features (e.g., temperature-changing masks) highlight the importance of sensory innovation in creating memorable user experiences.

At the same time, sustainability has become a key driver in sensory evaluation. This has led to the development of biodegradable textures, plant-based fragrances, and minimalist packaging, all designed to deliver an appealing sensory experience while reducing environmental impact. Additionally, the rise of neurocosmetics—a field that explores the connection between sensory stimulation and emotional well-being—has brought a new dimension to product development. Products are now being designed to elicit specific emotional responses, such as relaxation, confidence, or invigoration, through carefully curated sensory profiles.

The historical evolution of sensory evaluation in cosmetics showcases a journey from artisanal craftsmanship to cutting-edge science, reflecting the industry's dedication to merging tradition, innovation, and consumer-centricity. This continuous evolution ensures that cosmetics not only meet functional needs but also deliver meaningful, multisensory experiences that resonate with diverse audiences.

2. Sensory perception in cosmetics

The science of sensory modalities refers to the study of the different ways humans and animals perceive and process information from their environment through sensory organs. These modalities are the specific senses that allow us to interact with the world, including vision, hearing, touch, taste, and smell, as well as the proprioception or the vestibular sense. The neurological pathways of sensory perception involve complex interactions between the sensory organs, the brain, and the nervous system. Each sensory modality follows distinct neural pathways to generate sensory experiences, and these pathways significantly influence emotional responses and cognitive processes. In particular, the olfactory system (sense of smell) plays a unique role in shaping emotions, as it is directly linked to brain areas involved in memory, emotion, and behavior [5].

The diagram above (**Figure 5**) illustrates the sensory pathways. It highlights the journey of sensory information from initial stimulus detection (e.g., smell, sight, or sound) through sensory receptors, nerves, and key brain regions involved in emotional processing, such as the limbic system and the prefrontal cortex, ultimately reaching the brain's reward center (including the nucleus accumbens and ventral tegmental area).

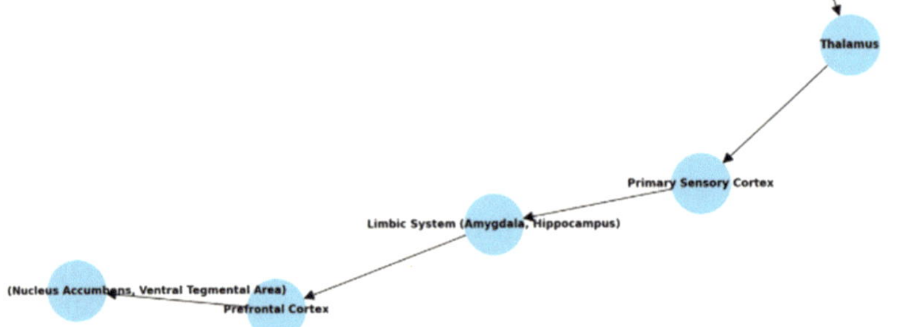

Figure 5.
Sensory pathways linking perception to the brain's reward center.

Each modality involves complex biological and neural processes, and the study of these modalities encompasses various fields such as neuroscience, psychology, cognitive science, and technology where sensory modalities are increasingly important in fields such as virtual reality, robotics, and human-computer interaction, in which multisensory experiences are engineered for immersive applications.

This is also known as multisensory integration, which allows individuals to perceive more than just isolated sensory data but a unified understanding of their surroundings. Understanding sensory modalities is crucial for developing therapeutic approaches in areas such as pain management, sensory disorders, and neurodegenerative diseases, and it also plays a role in the development of consumer products like cosmetics and dermatological treatments, where sensory experiences are integral [6].

2.1 The touch

Texture, consistency and spreadability are key attributes that influence how a product feels when applied to the skin, and they play an important role in consumer satisfaction and product performance.

- Texture refers to the physical feel of a product when applied to the skin, including its smoothness, grittiness, or creaminess. The texture of a cosmetic product can greatly influence its appeal. For example, oil-based products often have a heavier, more moisturizing texture, while gel-based products feel lighter and more refreshing. Viscosity refers to the thickness or flow resistance of a product. Higher-viscosity products, like creams and lotions, tend to have a denser texture, while lower-viscosity products, like serums or gels, feel more fluid.

- Consistency refers to the uniformity of the product's texture and the ease with which it can be applied. It ensures that the product applies evenly to the skin and delivers the intended effect without clumping, separating, or becoming uneven. A well-balanced emulsion will have a smooth and stable consistency. Ingredients like thickeners (e.g., xanthan gum, carbomers) and emulsifiers (e.g., lecithin, cetearyl alcohol) help control consistency by preventing separation and ensuring uniformity.

- Spreadability refers to how easily a product can be spread over the skin without resistance or pulling. Good spreadability enhances the user experience by making the product easy to apply and ensuring even coverage. Products with a smoother texture and more fluid consistency tend to spread effortlessly. Ingredients like silicones (dimethicone, cyclopentasiloxane) and natural oils (jojoba, almond oil) improve spreadability by reducing friction and helping the product glide on the skin.

Of course, the user's skin type also plays a role. The smooth texture of a high-quality product may provide feelings of comfort and indulgence, while an unpleasant texture may lead to dissatisfaction or product rejection. The combination of texture, consistency, and spreadability directly affects how consumers perceive a product's sensory appeal. In contrast, a rich, thick cream might appeal to those looking for intense hydration and a more luxurious experience. The sensory aspects of touch in cosmetics also evoke emotional responses. The smooth texture of a high-quality product may provide feelings of comfort and indulgence, while an unpleasant texture may lead to dissatisfaction or product rejection.

That is why the practical applications in product development can be:

- Formulation adjustments: Cosmetic formulators use various techniques to achieve the desired texture, consistency, and spreadability [7]. For example, adding different types of oils or adjusting the amount of thickening agents can modify how a product feels on the skin.

- Consumer testing: Product developers often perform sensory evaluation studies to assess the touch characteristics of products. These studies help identify consumer preferences and ensure the product delivers a satisfying sensory experience [8].

- Packaging: The type of packaging also influences the perceived texture and spreadability. For instance, airless pumps and jars allow consumers to easily dispense the product without waste, maintaining the consistency of the formula.

2.2 The sight

In cosmetics, sight plays a crucial role in the overall appeal of a product. Color, gloss, and visual appeal are key elements that not only influence consumer choice but also affect how the product is perceived in terms of quality, effectiveness, and desirability.

- Color in cosmetics refers to the shade, hue, and intensity of a product. It can include the color of the product itself (e.g., lipstick, foundation, eyeshadow) as well as the color it imparts to the skin. The color of a cosmetic product is one of the first attributes consumers notice. It has a significant impact on product perception, often influencing purchase decisions based on personal preferences, trends, and cultural associations.

    o Pigments and dyes: The color of a product is determined by the pigments (such as iron oxides, titanium dioxide, and mica) or dyes used in the formulation. The choice of pigments affects the final color and its intensity.

    o Skin Tone Matching: Products like foundations, concealers, and blushes are designed to complement a wide range of skin tones. The right color match enhances the natural beauty of the skin and provides a more flawless appearance [9].

    o Trends and cultural influence: Color trends in cosmetics often change based on seasonal shifts, fashion, and cultural movements. For instance, warm tones may be popular in the fall, while vibrant or pastel colors are favored in the spring and summer.

The color of a cosmetic product can evoke different emotions and associations. For example, bold red lipstick may be associated with confidence and empowerment, while soft pink shades may convey femininity and delicacy.

- Gloss refers to the shine or luster that a cosmetic product imparts on the skin or lips. It is a key visual characteristic in products like lip gloss, moisturizers, and highlighters. Gloss enhances the esthetic appeal of a product by making the skin or lips look healthier, more vibrant, and moisturized. It is often associated with youthful, dewy skin and a radiant, glowing complexion.

- o Ingredients: The glossiness of a product is influenced by ingredients such as oils (e.g., castor oil, jojoba oil), silicones (e.g., dimethicone, cyclopentasiloxane), and waxes. These ingredients help create a shiny finish while providing smoothness and moisture.

- o Formulation type: Gloss is often a key characteristic in products like lip glosses, highlighters, and certain skincare products (e.g., serums and moisturizers). A high-gloss finish is often sought after in products that aim to give a dewy, fresh appearance.

- o Matte vs. glossy: While gloss is desirable in some products (like lip gloss), other products may focus on achieving a matte finish, such as matte lipsticks or foundations. The contrast between matte and glossy products offers consumers a range of visual experiences and finishes. Glossy products are often perceived as more hydrating and youthful, as they reflect light and make the skin appear plump and moisturized. On the other hand, a matte finish may be favored for a more sophisticated, long-lasting, or oil-controlling effect.

- Visual appeal refers to the overall attractiveness of the cosmetic product in terms of color, packaging, texture, and finish. It is the cumulative effect of how a product looks both in the packaging and when applied to the skin. It plays a critical role in consumer attraction and purchasing decisions. It encompasses the esthetics of the product's design, including how it looks on the shelf, how it appears when applied, and how it fits into the user's beauty routine.

    - o Packaging design of a cosmetic product often contributes significantly to its visual appeal. Elegant, modern, or luxurious packaging can attract consumers and signal the quality of the product. For example, sleek glass containers, minimalist designs, and unique shapes are all factors that contribute to the appeal.

    - o Consistency is how a product appears in the packaging versus how it looks when applied. A foundation that appears one color in the bottle but applies much lighter or darker than expected may cause dissatisfaction.

    - o Shimmer, sheen, and finish: Products with shimmer or sheen, like highlighters or eyeshadows, can add an extra layer of visual appeal. These products create dimension and depth, enhancing the overall esthetic of makeup [10].

The visual appeal of a product is tied to consumer expectations. For instance, a high-quality lipstick that glides on smoothly and provides an even color payoff will have strong visual appeal, leading to a more positive experience and increased likelihood of repurchase.

Practical applications in product development:

- Color matching: Formulators often use color theory and skin tone research to develop products that complement a wide range of users. For example, foundations come in various shades to match different skin tones, while blushes and bronzers are designed to add natural warmth and dimension.

- Formulation adjustments for gloss: Cosmetic formulators balance gloss with other attributes such as longevity and comfort. For example, lip glosses might be made with ingredients that provide both shine and hydration without being too sticky or heavy.

- Consumer testing: Visual appeal is often evaluated through consumer testing to assess how products look on different skin types and how they hold up over time. Product developers consider factors like color payoff, gloss intensity, and finish when refining formulations.

- Marketing and branding: The visual presentation of a product in advertisements and on retail shelves is designed to attract attention. Packaging design, color schemes, and visual textures all play a role in creating a strong brand identity and appeal to the target market.

The sight aspect of cosmetics—color, gloss, and visual appeal—is fundamental to how products are perceived and experienced by consumers. Formulating products with the right color, gloss, and visual appeal can elevate the user experience, enhance satisfaction, and drive brand loyalty.

2.3 Smell

In cosmetics, smell plays a powerful role in the overall sensory experience and can significantly influence consumer satisfaction and emotional responses. Fragrance design is a crucial element that enhances the appeal of products, and its emotional impact can create lasting impressions and drive brand loyalty. It involves the creation of a scent profile that enhances the product's appeal and aligns with the brand's identity. This process includes selecting and blending different fragrance notes to create a pleasant and cohesive scent. A well-designed fragrance can elevate the user experience by making the product feel more luxurious, soothing, or invigorating. Fragrance design also helps to differentiate products in the market, as scent is often a key factor in consumer decision-making.

Fragrance is typically composed of three layers or "notes" that are released over time. The initial scent that is noticed immediately upon application is called the top notes. These are usually light, fresh, and citrusy, such as lemon, bergamot, or mint. Middle notes (Heart notes) develop after the top notes fade and form the core of the fragrance. Floral, fruity, or spicy notes, such as rose, lavender, or jasmine, are commonly used in this layer. Base notes are the lingering scent that lasts the longest. These notes are often deep and rich, such as vanilla, musk, or sandalwood.

Synthetic vs. natural ingredients is an important decision. Fragrances can be created using synthetic compounds (e.g., aldehydes, musks) or natural essential oils (e.g., lavender, citrus). The choice between synthetic and natural ingredients affects both the scent profile and the product's appeal to consumers with different preferences (e.g., those seeking natural, organic products) [11].

Some consumers may have sensitivities or allergies to certain fragrance ingredients. Fragrance-free or hypoallergenic formulations are often designed for individuals with sensitive skin or allergies. The fragrance is often tailored to suit the purpose of the product and the target market. For example, calming lavender scents are commonly used in skincare products designed for relaxation, while fresh citrus fragrances might be favored in products intended for an energizing or refreshing effect.

The emotional impact of a fragrance is deeply connected to the brain's limbic system, which processes emotions, memories, and behavior. The response triggered by fragrance is a key reason why scent plays such an important role in cosmetics. A fragrance can evoke feelings of relaxation, confidence, nostalgia, or energy, influencing how a person feels and interacts with the product. Scent is strongly linked to memory. This emotional connection can enhance the user experience and foster brand loyalty.

Fragrances are often designed to have specific emotional effects on the user:

- Relaxing scents: Floral or woody scents like lavender, chamomile, and sandalwood are often used in products aimed at reducing stress and promoting relaxation.

- Energizing scents: Citrus scents like lemon, orange, or grapefruit are often used in products that aim to energize and invigorate the user.

- Romantic or sensual scents: Warm, spicy, and musky notes (e.g., vanilla, amber, patchouli) are often used in perfumes and cosmetics that seek to evoke feelings of romance, sensuality, or allure.

Different cultures may have varying preferences for certain fragrances, which can influence emotional responses. For example, some cultures associate floral scents with femininity, while others may associate woody or spicy scents with masculinity. Beyond the emotional impact, fragrance can also contribute to a sense of well-being.

Fragrance in product development has some key points:

- Personalization: Customization of fragrance is becoming more popular in cosmetics, where consumers can choose scents that align with their personal preferences. Brands are also increasingly offering fragrance-free or lightly scented products to cater to sensitive consumers.

- Longevity: In cosmetics, the longevity of fragrance is important. For example, a fragrance in a skincare product should last long enough to create a pleasant experience but not overpower the user. On the other hand, in perfumes, the scent's longevity is often a key selling point.

- Sustainability and ethics: As consumers become more conscious of sustainability, there is growing interest in natural, ethically sourced fragrances. Companies are developing eco-friendly and cruelty-free fragrance options to meet consumer demand for products that align with their values.

- Fragrance testing: To ensure a positive emotional impact, fragrance testing is conducted to assess how different scents are perceived by a target audience. This helps ensure that the fragrance enhances the product's effectiveness and appeal [12].

Fragrance can be used as a marketing tool using different strategies. Many brands use signature scents as part of their branding. For instance, certain fragrances can evoke the feeling of luxury or relaxation, which becomes synonymous with the brand's identity. The way a fragrance is presented can influence how it's perceived. A beautifully designed bottle or jar, along with the fragrance, can create a sensory experience that makes the product more memorable. Brands often use fragrance to connect emotionally with their audience. For example, a skincare brand might use a calming lavender scent to evoke relaxation and self-care, while a fragrance brand might use warm, exotic notes to create an air of sophistication and mystery.

The smell of a cosmetic product, created through careful fragrance design, is a powerful tool that influences the emotional response of consumers. As a result, fragrance design is a key component of product development in the cosmetics industry, impacting consumer satisfaction, brand loyalty, and even product efficacy.

2.4 The sound

In cosmetics, sound is a less obvious but still significant sensory modality that contributes to the overall user experience. Auditory cues during product application—such as the sound of sprays, emulsions, or the subtle noise produced when applying creams and lotions—can influence perceptions of product quality, effectiveness, and enjoyment.

- Sprays and mists refer to products that are dispensed as a fine aerosol or liquid spray, such as facial mists, body sprays, deodorants, and perfume. The sound produced when spraying a product can influence the perception of the product's texture, effectiveness, and luxury. A smooth, continuous, and soft "mist" sound is often associated with a high-quality product. For example, facial mists with a fine spray nozzle produce a light, gentle sound that suggests an even and delicate application. The hissing sound made when a product is sprayed (e.g., in deodorants or hairsprays) can convey a sense of freshness, activation, or even efficiency. A loud or forceful spray might suggest a more powerful product, while a softer spray might imply gentleness and refinement. The sound of a spray or mist can be refreshing and invigorating, adding to the sensory experience of feeling "spritzed" or revitalized. It can also enhance the feeling of freshness, which is why many face mists and body sprays emphasize a cooling, energizing sound.

- Emulsions refer to products that have a creamy or gel-like consistency, typically consisting of a blend of oil and water. Examples include moisturizers, lotions, and gels. The sound produced when applying emulsions can be subtle but plays a role in the perceived texture and quality of the product. The gentle sound of cream or lotion being rubbed onto the skin can be perceived as soothing [13]. A smooth, non-squeaky sound during application suggests that the product is gliding on easily, providing a pleasant tactile experience. The sound of a product being absorbed into the skin (e.g., a light "squelch" or "soak-in" noise) can convey the product's effectiveness. A satisfying, quiet absorption can suggest that the product is being quickly absorbed, leaving the skin soft and non-greasy. A subtle sound can also indicate the consistency of the product. Thicker creams might produce a slightly "thicker" or "heavier" sound when being spread across the skin, while lighter lotions or gels may have a more fluid, airy sound.

- Products like facial cleansers, exfoliating scrubs, and cleansing foams are applied to the skin for cleaning or exfoliating purposes. The sound of the product in action, such as a foaming cleanser or scrub, can influence the perceived effectiveness and sensory enjoyment of the product.

    - Foaming sounds: The gentle bubbling or foaming sound when a cleanser is massaged ointo the skin can convey freshness and a deep cleansing experience. It's often associated with a product that is working actively to cleanse the skin.

    - Scrubbing sounds: Exfoliating products with granular textures may produce a soft, granular "scratching" or "scrubbing" sound when massaged onto the skin. This sound can evoke a sense of exfoliation and removal of dead skin cells, contributing to the feeling of smoothness and rejuvenation.

    - Squeaky clean: After using a cleanser or exfoliant, some users may notice a subtle "squeak" when they run their fingers over the skin, indicating that the skin is clean and free from excess oil. This sound can enhance the feeling of cleanliness and refreshment.

The sound of the product being dispensed from its packaging can also contribute to the overall auditory experience. The noise produced when opening or dispensing a product can influence the perception of quality. For example, a well-designed pump or tube that dispenses a product with a satisfying "click" or "squirt" can suggest precision and convenience. The sound of opening a jar or unscrewing a cap or lid can signal a premium product. A smooth, quiet twist or snap can indicate a well-made, secure container, which in turn influences how consumers perceive the product's value. Airless pumps, often used for sensitive products like serums, can produce a subtle "whoosh" or "suction" sound when dispensed. This sound can reinforce the idea of product protection and freshness [14].

Some cosmetic products are applied by tapping or patting onto the skin, such as serums, eye creams, or foundations. The rhythmic tapping sound can evoke a sense of care, precision, and delicacy in application. A soft tapping sound, such as when applying a lightweight serum, often conveys a gentle, calming effect. This type of application is frequently associated with soothing products that require a delicate touch. The sound of tapping may also be perceived as part of the product's performance. For example, tapping on a foundation or concealer can signal the need for even distribution and blending, contributing to the perception of a smooth, flawless finish. Auditory cues engage the user's senses more holistically, enhancing their connection to the product. For instance, the combination of sight, touch, and sound during product application can create a more immersive and satisfying experience.

The sound of a product can evoke a specific emotional response. For example, a light misting sound can be refreshing and energizing, making it ideal for morning skincare routines. Conversely, the soothing sound of tapping or gentle application can create a calming, meditative experience, perfect for evening skincare rituals. Auditory cues, such as the sound of a spray nozzle or the smooth application of an emulsion, can contribute to the overall perception of product quality. High-quality products often produce more refined and pleasing sounds during application, which can reinforce the idea of luxury and attention to detail.

The sound of a cosmetic product during application—whether it's the gentle spray of a mist, the subtle squelch of a cream being absorbed, or the rhythmic tapping

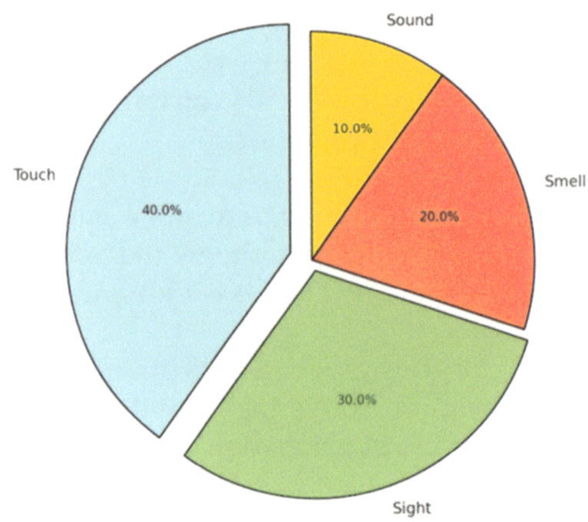

Figure 6.
The relationship between sensory modalities and their influence on consumer perception.

of a serum—plays a significant role in shaping the user experience. Auditory cues can influence perceptions of product quality, effectiveness, and emotional impact, contributing to a more immersive and satisfying beauty routine. Sound, in combination with other sensory modalities like sight, touch, and smell, helps create a holistic experience that can strengthencisfaction and loyalty (**Figure 6**).

3. Influence of culture and personal experiences

The psychology of sensory preferences is deeply influenced by culture and personal experiences, both of which shape how individuals perceive and respond to sensory stimuli such as sight, sound, smell, taste, and touch. In the context of cosmetics, these preferences are essential for understanding how different sensory elements—such as fragrance, texture, and color—are received by consumers across various cultural backgrounds and personal histories.

3.1 The cultural influence on sensory preferences

Culture plays a pivotal role in shaping how individuals perceive and interpret sensory stimuli. Different cultures have distinct associations with sensory experiences, which can influence preferences for certain textures, fragrances, colors, and sounds in cosmetics.

- Fragrance preferences: In many Western cultures, fresh and light scents like citrus or floral notes are commonly preferred, often linked to cleanliness and vitality. Conversely, in Eastern cultures, warm, spicy, and woody scents (e.g., sandalwood, jasmine, or incense) are often favored, symbolizing tradition, spirituality, and relaxation. For example, in some Middle Eastern cultures, oud (a rich, woody fragrance) is highly revered and is often used in perfumes and cosmetic products. The cultural attachment to specific scents can influence how a person perceives and enjoys fragrances in products like skincare, body lotions, and perfumes. In Japanese culture, the concept of "wabi-sabi" emphasizes subtlety and simplicity, leading to a preference for light, understated fragrances in cosmetics. On the other hand, in Latin American cultures, vibrant and bold scents might be more appreciated, reflecting the lively and colorful cultural ethos.

- Texture preferences: Different cultures also have varying preferences for textures in skincare and cosmetic products. In Asian cultures, lightweight, gel-like, or watery textures are often preferred, as they are perceived as more refreshing and suited to warmer climates. In contrast, Western cultures might lean toward thicker, creamier textures, associating them with moisturizing and anti-aging benefits. In hotter and more humid regions, such as Southeast Asia, people tend to favor lighter textures that are easily absorbed and non-greasy. In colder climates, such as in Northern Europe or North America, richer and more emollient textures (like balms and heavy creams) are preferred for their moisturizing properties in harsh winters.

- Color preferences: Cultural symbolism can influence the appeal of certain colors in cosmetic products. For example, in Western cultures, shades of red and pink are often associated with beauty, femininity, and passion, leading to their prevalence in makeup products like lipsticks and blushes. In Asian cultures, colors like peach, coral, and nude are more commonly preferred, often seen as soft and natural. During cultural festivals or special occasions, certain colors might become more popular. For instance, red is considered auspicious in many Asian cultures, leading to its frequent use in cosmetics during holidays or celebrations like the Chinese New Year or Diwali.

- Taste and eating habits: Cultural preferences in food can also extend to sensory experiences in cosmetics. For instance, in cultures where sweet, rich, and spicy flavors are common in cuisine (e.g., Indian or Middle Eastern cultures), there might be a greater affinity for sweet or spicy-scented skincare products. Conversely, in cultures with a preference for fresh or savory flavors (e.g., Mediterranean cultures), light, fresh scents may be more appealing.

3.2 Personal experiences and sensory preferences

Personal experiences are unique to each individual and can significantly influence how they perceive and enjoy sensory experiences. These experiences can stem from past events, memories, individual tastes, and even personal health conditions.

- Past experiences and memories: Personal memories linked to specific scents, textures, or colors can influence an individual's sensory preferences. For example, if a person associates the scent of lavender with positive childhood memories of visiting their grandmother's house, they may have a heightened preference for lavender in cosmetics as an adult. Fragrances and textures can trigger specific emotional responses based on past experiences. For example, a person who has experienced stress or anxiety may prefer soothing lavender or chamomile fragrances because of their association with relaxation and calmness. Conversely, someone who associates a particular scent with an unpleasant memory might avoid it in cosmetics.

- Health and skin sensitivities: Personal health conditions, such as allergies to specific ingredients or skin sensitivities, can influence preferences for certain textures or scents. People with sensitive skin may prefer fragrance-free or hypoallergenic products with gentle textures that are less likely to irritate. An individual's skin type (e.g., oily, dry, sensitive) can also influence their texture preferences. For instance, people with dry skin may prefer richer, more emollient textures like creams or balms, while those with oily skin may lean toward lightweight gels or serums that absorb quickly and do not leave a greasy residue.

- Psychological factors: Personal preferences often lean toward products that feel comfortable and familiar. For example, someone who grew up using a specific type of soap or body lotion may continue to prefer those products throughout their life due to a sense of nostalgia or comfort. Familiarity with certain scents, textures, or colors can enhance a person's sense of security and trust in a product. Cosmetics also serve as a form of self-expression, and personal experiences can shape how individuals choose products to reflect their identity. For instance, someone who values individuality may gravitate toward bold and unique colors in makeup, while someone with a preference for subtlety might favor neutral tones.

- Social influence: Personal experiences are often shaped by social interactions and societal norms. A person may be influenced by family members, peers, or celebrities in their choice of cosmetic products. Social trends and the influence of beauty standards can drive individual preferences, especially when it comes to makeup, fragrance, and skincare products that align with current beauty ideals.

In today's globalized world, many individuals are exposed to multiple cultures and experiences, leading to hybrid preferences. For example, a person raised in a Western culture but living in an Asian country may develop a unique set of sensory preferences, blending the influences of both cultures. This could manifest in their skincare routine, such as a preference for light textures (influenced by Asian beauty trends) combined with a fondness for floral fragrances (common in Western cosmetics). As people move between cultures, they may adopt new sensory preferences while maintaining some from their original culture. This process, known as acculturation, can lead to changes in fragrance or texture preferences over time as individuals adapt to new surroundings and cultural influences.

A heatmap is a powerful tool for brands to visualize the complex relationships between sensory attributes and consumer preferences. It helps guide product development, formulation adjustments, and targeted marketing strategies by highlighting which sensory characteristics are the most important to each consumer segment (**Figure** 7).

The color scale reflects the preference scores, where warmer colors (reds/oranges) represent higher preferences and cooler colors (blues) represent lower preferences. This visualization allows for an easy comparison of how each group perceives different sensory attributes of a skincare cream.

The psychology of sensory preferences is deeply intertwined with culture and personal experiences. Cultural norms, traditions, and symbolism influence how individuals perceive and react to different sensory stimuli, while personal memories, health conditions, and social factors further shape these preferences. In the context of cosmetics, understanding the role of culture and personal experiences in shaping sensory preferences is crucial for developing products that resonate with diverse consumer bases and enhance their overall experience.

DOI: http://dx.doi.org/10.5772/intechopen.1009804

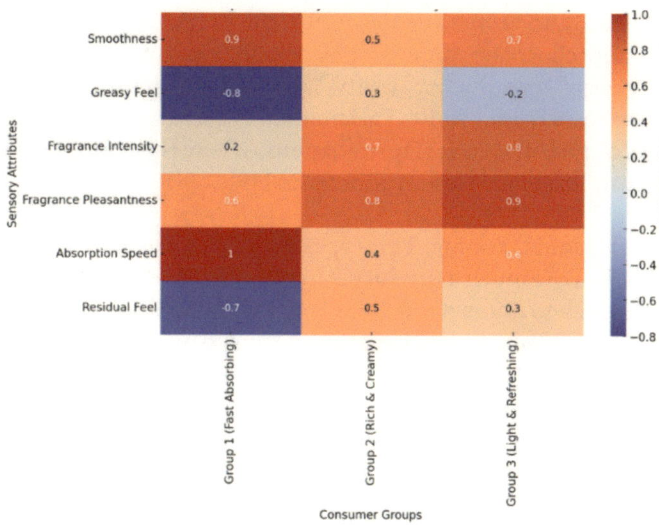

Figure 7.
Heatmap based on the sensory preference data for the three consumer groups and various sensory attributes.

4. Methodologies in sensory evaluation

4.1 Subjective evaluation

This method of sensory testing involves human participants who assess products based on their personal experiences, perceptions, and preferences. This type of evaluation is inherently qualitative, as it relies on individual judgment and sensory responses.

- Sensory panels:

  a. Expert panels are used to evaluate specific sensory attributes that require high levels of training and expertise. For example, in the food industry, a trained expert panel might assess the texture, mouthfeel, and aroma of a new type of snack. A panel of trained wine tasters evaluates the aroma, flavor profile, and mouthfeel of different wines. The experts provide detailed feedback on the nuances of taste and texture, such as "fruity," "tannic," or "smooth." In the cosmetic industry, experts might evaluate the spreadability, absorbency, and feel of a new skincare product.

  b. Consumer panels: These panels are composed of everyday consumers who reflect the target market. Consumer panels provide feedback based on their preferences, allowing brands to assess whether their product will be well-received by the general population. A consumer panel might be asked to rate different types of shampoo based on factors such as scent, ease of use, and hair softness. For a new deodorant, consumer panels could provide valuable feedback on scent longevity, skin irritation, and overall satisfaction.

- Sensory tests:

  a. Descriptive analysis helps to identify and quantify the sensory characteristics of a product. Panelists are trained to detect subtle differences in attributes like flavor, texture, and aroma and describe them in specific terms. In the development of a new chocolate, for example, panelists might describe its flavor as "bitter," "sweet," "creamy," or "fruity" and rate the intensity of each characteristic on a scale from 1 to 10. This method is useful in evaluating the sensory properties of pharmaceutical formulations, where the texture or flavor of a medicine can influence patient adherence [15].

b. Affective (Hedonic) testing: This type of testing focuses on consumer preferences, that is, how much a product is liked or disliked. It is typically used in market research to understand consumer reactions to a product. A company might conduct a hedonic test for a new beverage by asking consumers to rate it on a scale from 1 (dislike extremely) to 9 (like extremely). Cosmetic companies often use hedonic tests to assess the overall satisfaction with products like lotions or creams. For example, they may ask participants to rate the overall feel and appearance of their skin after using a product.

c. Discrimination testing: Discrimination tests are used to determine if there is a significant difference between two or more products in terms of sensory characteristics. A triangle test might be used to see if consumers can identify which of the two sodas has a higher level of sweetness. In the fragrance industry, a discrimination test might be used to determine whether consumers can distinguish between two similar scents, or if a new formulation has a different scent profile.

d. Rating scales:

- o Unstructured scales: These scales allow panelists to provide qualitative feedback, such as descriptive words or phrases, rather than quantifying their responses. For a new perfume, panelists may be asked to describe the scent in their own words, using descriptors like "floral," "woody," or "spicy." Unstructured feedback is commonly used in exploratory product development when the goal is to capture initial impressions and broad sensory experiences.Structured scales: Structured scales allow for more precise measurements, often on a numeric or Likert-type scale, where panelists rate products on specific attributes (e.g., sweetness, texture, satisfaction) [16]. In a test of hand creams, panelists might rate the product's "smoothness" on a 1–5 scale (1 = very rough, 5 = very smooth). Structured scales are commonly used in both product development and consumer satisfaction surveys.

e. Test procedures

- o Monadic testing: In monadic testing, each product is tested independently, and participants give feedback on each product in isolation. This is useful for assessing the individual qualities of each product without direct comparison. A participant might test one brand of toothpaste and provide feedback on its flavor, texture, and overall satisfaction. Monadic testing is often used when a company wants to understand how a single product performs in the market.

- Paired comparison testing: In this testing, two products are tested simultaneously, and participants are asked to choose the one they prefer or identify which product has a stronger attribute. In a coffee brand comparison, participants might be given two samples and asked to select which one has a stronger coffee flavor. This type of test is used when companies want to compare two competing products in a direct head-to-head comparison.

- Ranking tests: In ranking tests, participants are asked to rank multiple products based on a specific criterion, such as preference, aroma, or taste. Participants might be given three different lip balms and asked to rank them from best to worst based on smoothness, scent, and texture. Ranking tests are useful when evaluating multiple products and identifying which one is the most preferred in a given category.

f. Control of bias

- Randomization: This ensures that product presentation order does not influence results. For example, in a taste test, participants might be given samples in a random order to prevent one sample from being preferred simply because it was presented first.

- Blinding: In double-blind tests, neither the participant nor the evaluator knows which product is being tested. This prevents biases from affecting the results.

- Environmental control: Sensory testing is often done in controlled environments to eliminate distractions (e.g., temperature, lighting, or odors) that might influence a participant's sensory experience.

g. Data analysis

- Statistical methods: Data from subjective evaluation are often analyzed using methods like ANOVA (Analysis of Variance) to assess if there are significant differences between products or groups. Post-hoc tests might be used to identify which specific groups differ.

- Sensory profiles: These are developed by analyzing the data from descriptive analysis and can highlight the specific sensory strengths or weaknesses of a product. For example, a sensory profile might show that a specific lotion is highly rated for smoothness but has a lower score for scent.

In a real-world example, a new line of moisturizers is created. Experts in dermatology and cosmetic formulation might evaluate the product for texture, absorbency, and irritation potential. A broader group of consumers might rate their satisfaction with the product's fragrance, moisturizing effects, and skin feel. A triangle test could be used to determine if consumers can distinguish between two variations of the moisturizer (e.g., one with added SPF and one without). This method provides real-world consumer insights, allows for the assessment of emotional responses and personal preferences, and is useful for product development and market research, especially when targeting a specific demographic. However, results can be influenced by individual biases, mood, or environmental factors, and larger sample sizes are often required to obtain statistically significant results. By combining these methods, companies can ensure that their products are both scientifically sound and well-received by consumers.

4.2 Instrumental methods

Instrumental methods refer to the use of various devices and instruments to objectively measure the sensory attributes of a product, complementing or sometimes replacing subjective human evaluation. These methods are often more precise and can provide reproducible data. They are typically used to measure physical properties like texture, color, viscosity, and aroma, which are then correlated with human sensory responses.

a. Texture analysis measures the texture properties of a product, such as hardness, chewiness, smoothness, or stickiness, which are important for food, cosmetic, and pharmaceutical products. The texture analyzer is a device that measures the force required to deform or compress a product, such as a food item or a cosmetic cream. It can be used to evaluate parameters like hardness, springiness, cohesiveness, and adhesiveness. In the food industry, a texture analyzer might be used to measure the firmness of a piece of fruit or the crispiness of a snack. In cosmetics, it can be used to evaluate the spreadability or thickness of lotions and creams.

b. Color measurement provides objective, quantitative measurements of color attributes, such as hue, saturation, and lightness (brightness). This is particularly useful in products like food, cosmetics, and textiles, where color is an important factor. Colorimeter measures the color of a product using standard color spaces (e.g., CIELAB or RGB). The instrument provides numerical values for color characteristics. In cosmetics, a colorimeter can be used to assess the consistency of the color in a batch of foundation or lipstick. A spectrophotometer measures the reflection or transmission of light across the spectrum, providing detailed color data. It can also measure gloss and translucency.

c. Viscosity measurement measures the flow behavior or thickness of a liquid, gel, or cream. Viscosity is an important parameter for products like sauces, lotions, and paints. The Viscometer is an instrument that measures the resistance of a fluid to flow. Different types include rotational viscometers, capillary viscometers, and falling ball viscometers. The rheometer measures the flow properties of more complex fluids, such as gels or emulsions, which exhibit both solid and liquid-like behavior. A rotational viscometer could be used to assess the viscosity of a shampoo or hand cream. In pharmaceuticals, viscosity measurement is used to evaluate the consistency of ointments or suspensions.

d. Aroma and volatile compound analysis measures the volatile compounds that contribute to a product's aroma. This is especially important for perfumes, food, and cosmetics. Gas chromatography (GC) separates and analyzes volatile compounds in a sample. When paired with a mass spectrometer (GC-MS), it can provide detailed information on the composition of aromas and flavors. In fragrance development, GC-MS can be used to identify the individual chemical compounds responsible for the scent of a perfume. Electronic Nose (E-nose) is a device that uses an array of sensors to detect and analyze odors, mimicking the human sense of smell. It provides rapid and reproducible results.

e. A pH meter can be used to measure the pH, or acidity, of a product, which can affect taste (for food) or stability (for cosmetics or pharmaceuticals). The device measures the concentration of hydrogen ions in a solution and provides an accurate pH value. Titration is a chemical method used to determine the acidity or alkalinity of a substance by adding a reagent until a reaction endpoint is reached. In the food industry, pH meters are commonly used to measure the acidity of fruit juices or sauces. In cosmetics, pH measurement ensures that products like shampoos or creams are skin-friendly and do not disrupt the skin's natural pH balance.

f. Optical density and transparency measurements show the clarity or opacity of a product. This is particularly important for products like beverages, gels, or lotions. A turbidimeter measures the degree of cloudiness or opacity in a liquid. A spectrophotometer can also be used to measure the transparency or absorbance of light through a sample, providing data on its clarity. In the beverage industry, a turbidimeter could be used to measure the clarity of fruit juices or soft drinks. In cosmetics, a spectrophotometer can be used to evaluate the transparency of facial serums or sunscreens.

g. Taste and flavor measurement: An electronic tongue mimics the human sense of taste, providing objective measurements of basic tastes (sweet, sour, salty, bitter, umami) and complex flavors. It is a sensor-based system that detects and analyzes the chemical components responsible for taste. In the food industry, an electronic tongue could be used to measure the bitterness or sweetness of a new soft drink formula. In pharmaceuticals, it could help in formulating better-tasting oral medications, such as syrups or chewable forms.

Instrumental methods provide reproducible and quantifiable data, reducing human error and bias. Instruments can detect subtle differences in product attributes that may not be easily perceived by human senses. Instrumental methods often require less time than subjective evaluation, especially for attributes like texture or color. While instrumental methods can measure objective properties, they do not always correlate directly with human sensory experiences. For example, a product might have the right texture based on instrument readings but still be perceived as unpleasant by consumers. Some instrumental methods, like gas chromatography or electronic noses, can be expensive and require specialized training to operate.

Integrative approaches in sensory evaluation combine both subjective (human) and objective (instrumental) methods to provide a comprehensive understanding of how consumers perceive a product's sensory attributes. These approaches aim to correlate human sensory experiences with instrumental measurements, enabling a more complete and accurate assessment of product characteristics. This approach is particularly useful when subjective evaluations alone may not provide sufficient insight into a product's sensory profile, or when it's necessary to validate human perceptions with objective measurements.

4.3 Combining subjective and instrumental data

In recent years, digital technologies and artificial intelligence (AI) have significantly advanced the field of sensory analysis. These innovations have revolutionized how sensory data are collected, analyzed, and applied, enabling faster, more accurate, and more comprehensive insights into consumer preferences and product performance. The integration of AI with sensory science has the potential to streamline product development, enhance consumer experience, and optimize sensory evaluation processes.

a. Digital sensory evaluation tools enable the capture, analysis, and interpretation of sensory data through online platforms and mobile apps, offering real-time feedback and making sensory evaluation more accessible.

- Online consumer panels: Companies can conduct sensory evaluations remotely, using digital platforms to collect consumer preferences, sensory ratings, and feedback on various product attributes. These platforms allow for global consumer participation, increasing the diversity of data.

- Mobile sensory apps: Apps allow consumers to rate products (e.g., food, beverages, cosmetics) based on sensory attributes like taste, smell, texture, and appearance. These apps use sensors embedded in smartphones to measure environmental factors (e.g., temperature, humidity) that could affect sensory perception.

Cosmetics companies gather feedback on product texture, fragrance, and overall experience through digital panels.

b. AI-powered sensory data analysis

AI and machine learning (ML) algorithms analyze large datasets from sensory tests, identifying patterns and correlations that might be difficult for humans to detect. This allows for deeper insights into consumer preferences and product attributes.

- Machine learning for pattern recognition: AI algorithms can be trained to recognize patterns in consumer feedback (e.g., preferences for specific flavors or textures) and correlate them with product characteristics (e.g., chemical composition, texture, or aroma).

- Predictive analytics: AI can predict consumer preferences and market trends based on historical data and sensory feedback. This helps in developing products that align with consumer expectations even before testing. In cosmetics, AI can help predict how different product formulations will be perceived by different demographic groups based on sensory profiles.

c. Virtual sensory reality (VSR) and augmented reality (AR) are emerging technologies that simulate sensory experiences, allowing users to experience a product's sensory attributes in a digital environment.

- Virtual sensory reality (VSR): VR technology can be used to simulate the experience of consuming or using a product. For example, a user could experience the taste or texture of a product through a VR headset paired with sensory stimulation devices (e.g., taste simulators).

- Augmented reality (AR): AR can be used to visualize product attributes, such as texture or color, in real-time by overlaying digital information onto physical objects. This allows consumers to experience a product's sensory attributes more interactively. In cosmetics and fragrances, AR technology is used in virtual try-on applications, allowing users to see how products like makeup or skincare items would look or feel on their skin before purchasing.

d. AI-driven sensory profiling and descriptive analysis

AI is now being used to automate sensory profiling, traditionally done by human experts, by analyzing data from sensory panels and providing detailed, quantitative sensory descriptions.

- Automated descriptive analysis: AI tools can process sensory data from consumer panels or trained sensory experts and generate detailed sensory profiles for products. This includes descriptors like "smooth," "creamy," or "crunchy" and can even quantify their intensity.

- Sensory attribute correlation: AI can correlate specific sensory attributes (e.g., texture, taste, aroma) with consumer preference scores, providing more accurate and actionable insights.

In cosmetics, AI analyzes how consumers describe sensory attributes (e.g., smoothness, fragrance, greasiness) and correlates these with ingredient combinations to help develop products that match consumer preferences.

e. Real-time sensory monitoring with digital sensors

Digital sensors are increasingly used to monitor sensory attributes in real-time, providing continuous data on product quality and performance during production or use.

- Electronic nose (E-nose): AI-powered E-nose devices are used to measure and analyze aromas in real-time, identifying and classifying odors. These devices are becoming more sophisticated, capable of detecting subtle differences in fragrance profiles.

- Electronic tongue (E-tongue): AI-enhanced E-tongue systems are used to analyze the taste of products by detecting the chemical compounds responsible for basic tastes (sweet, sour, salty, bitter, umami).

- Smart texture analyzers: These devices use AI algorithms to assess texture changes during the product's lifecycle, from production to consumer use, providing real-time insights into product consistency.

In cosmetic manufacturing, real-time monitoring of product texture and fragrance ensures quality control in cosmetic formulations.

f. Sentiment analysis for consumer feedback

AI-powered sentiment analysis tools analyze large volumes of consumer feedback from social media, reviews, and surveys to extract valuable insights into product perception and market trends.

- Natural language processing (NLP): NLP algorithms are used to analyze written or spoken feedback from consumers, identifying positive or negative sentiments related to sensory attributes such as taste, texture, or fragrance [17].

- Social media monitoring: AI tools track mentions of products on social media platforms and analyze consumer reactions to identify trends, preferences, and potential areas for improvement.

In Cosmetics sentiment analysis is used to track consumer reactions to new skincare products or fragrances.

g. Deep learning for sensory data integration

Deep learning algorithms are used to integrate sensory data from various sources (consumer panels, instrumental measurements, market data) and create more accurate predictive models of consumer preferences and product performance [18].

- Deep neural networks (DNNs): DNNs are used to analyze complex, high-dimensional sensory data, learning from both human feedback and instrumental measurements to predict how changes in product formulation will affect consumer satisfaction. For cosmetics, DNNs are used to refine product formulations based on the correlation between ingredient combinations and sensory perceptions

- AI-driven optimization: These models can optimize product formulations in real-time by predicting how specific ingredient changes (e.g., aroma compounds or texture modifiers) will influence consumer preferences.

AI tools can process large amounts of sensory data quickly, providing real-time insights and reducing the time needed for product development and testing. AI and digital tools provide more accurate and reproducible results, reducing the potential for human error in sensory evaluations. Digital and AI-based tools can reduce the need for physical testing by simulating sensory experiences or predicting outcomes, saving both time and money in product development. AI-based systems can scale easily to handle large datasets, enabling companies to analyze data from global consumer panels and product trials. AI can tailor sensory experiences to specific consumer preferences, allowing for the development of personalized products.

AI and digital systems are only as good as the data they are trained on. Poor-quality or biased data can lead to inaccurate predictions. Implementing AI-driven sensory analysis systems can be complex and require specialized expertise. While AI offers powerful tools, some consumers may be skeptical of AI-generated sensory analysis, preferring traditional human-based sensory evaluations.

AI and digital technologies are transforming sensory evaluation by enabling more precise, efficient, and scalable analysis of consumer preferences and product attributes. These advancements are making it possible to develop products that are better aligned with consumer expectations and improve the overall sensory experience.

5. Future trends in sensory science

5.1 Personalization in sensory experiences

The future of sensory science in cosmetics is moving toward hyper-personalization, where AI and data analytics tailor products to individual consumer preferences.

- AI-driven customization: Brands are now using AI to analyze consumer preferences and create personalized fragrances, textures, and formulations.

- Adaptive skincare: Some innovative products change their texture upon application, such as gel-to-cream formulations that activate upon skin contact.

- Microbiome-based customization: Advances in microbiome research allow brands to create products that adapt to an individual's skin chemistry, providing unique sensorial effects based on the user's biological profile.

Example: Lancôme's Le Teint Particulier foundation offers a customized texture and shade based on an individual's skin type and tone, using AI to fine-tune formulations.

5.2 Smart technologies in sensory evaluation

Innovations in sensory science are enhancing the way brands measure, predict, and optimize consumer experiences.

- Digital sensory testing: AI-driven models simulate how consumers perceive texture, scent, and visual appeal, allowing formulators to predict user satisfaction without requiring large-scale consumer trials.

- Haptic and multi-sensory packaging: The future of cosmetics may include temperature-sensitive or tactile-enhancing packaging to elevate the sensory experience (e.g., warming applicators for creams or vibrating applicators for serums).

- Wearable devices for sensory feedback: Emerging technologies in biosensors and wearables can track how a product interacts with the skin, measuring hydration, fragrance diffusion, and sensory longevity in real-time.

Some fragrance brands are developing AI-driven scent diffusers that adjust perfume intensity based on the wearer's body chemistry and external conditions.

5.3 Future trends in sensory-functionality optimization

a. Neurocosmetics: Sensory meets science:

Future formulations will incorporate neurocosmetic ingredients, designed to enhance mood and emotional well-being through sensory stimulation. Examples include dopamine-boosting fragrances, self-warming textures, and stress-reducing scents.

b. Customizable sensory profiles:

Advances in AI and biotechnology will allow consumers to customize product textures, scents, and colors based on individual preferences. Smart beauty devices will enable on-demand texture and sensory modifications for different climates and skin conditions.

c. Sustainable sensory innovation:

The next generation of sensory enhancers will be based on bio-engineered and biodegradable materials, ensuring luxurious feel without environmental harm. Future eco-friendly silicones and vegan sensory alternatives will maintain the appeal of traditional cosmetics while being planet-conscious.

6. Conclusion

As the beauty industry evolves, sensory science must navigate the complexities of balancing consumer desires, sustainability, and technological advancements. The future of cosmetics will focus on customization, ethical formulation, and smart technology, ensuring that products deliver both an engaging sensory experience and functional performance. Brands that innovate in these areas will gain a competitive edge, enhancing consumer satisfaction and fostering long-term brand loyalty.

Sensory appeal and product functionality are deeply interconnected in cosmetics, requiring constant innovation and scientific advancements to maintain both aspects. As consumer expectations evolve, the industry must focus on new formulation technologies, AI-driven personalization, and sustainable alternatives to create products that are both sensorially delightful and functionally effective.

AI-powered beauty advisors are set to revolutionize the beauty industry by providing hyper-personalized and emotionally resonant experiences. Through advanced data analytics, AI can offer consumers not just tailored skincare regimens but also holistic sensory experiences that encompass fragrance, texture, and emotional connection. As AI continues to evolve, it will enable brands to create products and experiences that not only meet consumers' practical needs but also foster deeper emotional engagement, enhancing overall brand loyalty.

Sensory appeal and product functionality must be carefully balanced through scientific advancements, ML-optimized formulation, and sustainable innovation. A cosmetic producer that masters this balance will enhance sales and public attachment while maintaining dermatological and environmental integrity.

Author details

Felicia Andrei
Faculty of Pharmacy, Department I, University of Medicine and Pharmacy, Timisoara, Romania

*Address all correspondence to: felicia.andrei@umft.ro

References

[1] Vieira GS, Lavarde M, Fréville V, Rocha-Filho PA, Pensé-Lhéritier AM. Combining sensory and texturometer parameters to characterize different type of cosmetic ingredients. International Journal of Cosmetic Science. 2020;**42**(2):156-166. DOI: 10.1111/ics.12598

[2] Boinbaser L, Parente ME, Castura JC, Ares G. Dynamic sensory characterization of cosmetic creams during application using temporal check-all-that-apply (TCATA) questions. Food Quality and Preference. 2015;**45**:33-40

[3] Varela P, Ares G. Sensory profiling, the blurred line between sensory and consumer science. A review of novel methods for product characterization. Food Research International. 2012;**48**(2):893-908

[4] Schifferstein HNJ. From salad to bowl: The role of sensory analysis in product experience research. Food Quality and Preference. 2010;**21**(8):1059-1067. ISSN 0950-3293. DOI: 10.1016/j.foodqual.2010.07.007

[5] Calixto LS, Maia Campos PMBG, Picard C, Savary G. Brazilian and French sensory perception of complex cosmetic formulations: A cross-cultural study. International Journal of Cosmetic Science. 2020;**42**(1):60-67. DOI: 10.1111/ics.12586. Epub 2020 Jan 8

[6] Gilbert L, Picard C, Savary G, Grisel M. Impact of polymers on texture properties of cosmetic emulsions: A methodological approach. Journal of Sensory Studies. 2012;**27**(5):392-402. DOI: 10.1111/joss.12001

[7] Kim J et al. The role of rheology in cosmetics research: A review. Korea Australia Rheology Journal. 2024;**36**(4):271-282. DOI: 10.1007/s13367-024-00108-y

[8] Fabbron-Appas CT, Pandey P, Parekh HS, Sales CC, Duque M, Andréo FN, et al. Impact of different emollient esters on body emulsions: Sensory, physicochemical, and biometrological characterization. Journal of Sensory Studies. 2021;**36**:4. DOI: 10.1111/joss.12660

[9] Kelchen M, Menon G, Ten Eyck P, Prettypaul D, Brogden NK. A pilot study to evaluate the effects of topically applied cosmetic creams on epidermal responses. Skin Pharmacology and Physiology. 2018;**31**(5):269-282. DOI: 10.1159/000490531

[10] Fabbron-Appas CT, Pandey P, Parekh HS, Sales CC, Duque M, Andréo FN, et al. Impact of different emollient esters on body emulsions: Sensory, physicochemical, and biometrological characterization. Journal of Sensory Studies. 2021;**36**:34. DOI: 10.1111/joss.12660

[11] Parente ME, Ares G, Manzoni AV. Application of two consumer profiling techniques to cosmetic emulsions. Journal of Sensory Studies. 2010;**25**(5):685-705. DOI: 10.1111/j.1745-459x.2010.00297.x

[12] Rico F, Mazabel A, Egurrola G, Pulido J, Barrios N, Marquez R, et al. Meta-analysis and analytical methods in cosmetics formulation: A review. Cosmetics. 2024;**11**(1):1. DOI: 10.3390/cosmetics11010001

[13] Franzol A, Banin TM, Brazil TR, Rezende MC. Textural analyses and artificial neural network as optimization tools to predict the sensory perception

of cosmetic emulsions. Journal of Sensory Studies. 2022;**37**:5. DOI: 10.1111/joss.12776

[14] Infante VHP et al. Influence of physical-mechanical properties on SPF in sunscreen formulations on ex vivo and in vivo skin. International Journal of Pharmaceutics. 2021;**598**:122-162. DOI: 10.1016/j.ijpharm.2021.120262

[15] Marque C, Pensé-Lhéritier A-M, Bacle I. Sensory methods for cosmetics evaluation. In: Nonfood Sensory Practices, Woodhead Publishing Series in Food Science, Technology and Nutrition. Vol. 5. Sawston, Cambridge: WP, Woodhead Publishing, Elsevier; 2022. pp. 169-196. DOI: 10.1016/B978-0-12-821939-3.00012-9

[16] Cyriac F, Xin YT, Chow PS, Macbeath C. Tactile friction and rheological studies to objectify sensory properties of topical formulations. Journal of Rheology. 2022;**66**(2):305-326. DOI: 10.1122/8.0000341

[17] Franzol A, Banin TM, Brazil TR, Rezende MC. Rheological analyses and artificial neural network as optimization tools to predict the sensory perception of cosmetic emulsions. Materials Research. 2021;**24**(6):12. DOI: 10.1590/1980-5373-MR-2021-0252

[18] Deubler G, Zhang C, Talavera MJ, Swaney-Stueve M. Sensory evaluation in the personal care space: A review. Journal of Sensory Studies. 2022;**37**(6):e12788. DOI: 10.1111/joss.12788

Chapter 3

Establishing an Evidence-Based System for Cosmetic Safety and Efficacy Evaluation

Li Ye, Jianhua Zhang, Tian Chen, Dongcui Li and Peng Shu

Abstract

In the era of the booming cosmetics industry, safety and efficacy evaluation have become crucial aspects in ensuring product quality and meeting consumer demands. The Chinese cosmetics market has witnessed rapid development. With an increasing emphasis on the safety and efficacy of cosmetics, a relatively comprehensive evaluation system has been gradually established. As pioneers in the cosmetics industry, Europe and the United States also possess mature and advanced experience in this regard. Based on years of work experience in the fields related to cosmetics safety and efficacy evaluation, the author of this chapter has summarized the characteristics of China, Europe, and the United States in this area. For safety evaluation, the entry points include cosmetics raw materials, packaging materials, chemistry and microbiology, as well as human testing. For efficacy evaluation, it is classified into categories such as cosmetics for freckle—removing and whitening, anti-hair loss, sun protection, anti-aging, and acne—treatment, repair, soothing, and those suitable for sensitive skin. By integrating the application of new AI technologies, this chapter presents a relatively scientific evidence-based system for cosmetics safety and efficacy evaluation to boost the high-quality development of the cosmetics industry.

Keywords: cosmetics, evidence - based system, safety assessment, efficacy evaluation, AI

1. Introduction

The evidence-based system, in simple terms, is a comprehensive decision-making framework that is founded on scientific research evidence, industry standards and regulations, consumer feedback and market data, as well as expert opinions and consensus. At its core, it involves systematically collecting, evaluating, and integrating information from multiple sources to provide reliable grounds for the safety and efficacy of cosmetics. This ensures that every stage of cosmetics, from research and development to production and sales, adheres to high-quality standards. There is a multi-faceted necessity for establishing an evidence-based system for the safety and efficacy of cosmetics. Firstly, for consumers, accurate information regarding the safety and efficacy of cosmetics is crucial for making informed purchasing decisions. The evidence-based system can offer objective and scientific evidence, assisting consumers in selecting cosmetics that are truly suitable, safe, and effective for them and preventing potential health risks associated with the use of inappropriate products. Secondly, from the perspective of industry development, the evidence-based system contributes to regulating the order of the cosmetics market. It encourages enterprises to pay more attention to product quality; conduct product research, development, and promotion based on scientific evidence; and reduce adverse phenomena such as false efficacy claims. This, in turn, enhances the credibility and competitiveness of the entire industry. Thirdly, at the regulatory level, the evidence-based system provides strong support for regulatory authorities in formulating policies and regulations and conducting market supervision. It enables regulatory decisions to be more scientific and rational, ensuring the healthy and stable operation of the cosmetics market. With the continuous development of the cosmetics industry and the escalating demands of consumers, establishing a complete evidence-based system for safety and efficacy has become an inevitable trend. It will lay a solid foundation for the sustainable development of the industry.

2. Construction of an evidence-based system for cosmetic safety

The cosmetics industry is continuously growing on a global scale, with new products and technologies emerging constantly, offering consumers a wider range of choices. However, the issue of cosmetic safety is increasingly drawing the attention of the public and regulatory authorities. The chemical substances contained in cosmetics may have an impact on human health. Therefore, ensuring the safety of cosmetics is crucial for protecting consumer health and maintaining the industry's credibility. The cosmetic safety evaluation system is an essential safeguard for the safe market entry of cosmetics, involving multiple aspects such as ingredient analysis, toxicological testing, and clinical trials. This paper will provide a detailed discussion on the construction principles, evaluation methods, and risk assessment of the cosmetic safety evaluation system [1, 2].

2.1 Principles of constructing the cosmetic safety evaluation system

2.1.1 Principle of scientificity

The construction of the cosmetic safety evaluation system must be based on scientific principles and methods to ensure the accuracy and reliability of the evaluation results. Generally speaking, cosmetic safety assessment should follow the principle of weight of evidence, based on existing scientific data and relevant information, and adhere to the principles of science, fairness, transparency, and case-by-case analysis. During the implementation process, the independence of the safety assessment work should be guaranteed [3].

2.1.2 Principle of comprehensiveness

The evaluation system should cover all safety issues of cosmetics, including the safety of raw materials, risk substances, formulations, production processes, and packaging materials. This means that the evaluation system needs to take into account all aspects of cosmetics to ensure a comprehensive assessment of their safety. Moreover, cosmetic enterprises should have the concept of full life cycle safety assessment and risk management. That is to say, safety assessment should start before product development, be implemented at the time of product registration and filing, accompany the product after it goes to market, and run through the entire life cycle of the product [4, 5].

2.1.3 Principle of dynamism

With the development of science and technology and the changes in consumer demand, the cosmetic safety evaluation system should be continuously updated and improved. This requires the evaluation system to adapt to new scientific discoveries and technological progress, as well as the new requirements of consumers for the safety of cosmetics.

2.1.4 Principle of international coordination

Considering the global circulation of cosmetics, the evaluation system should be consistent with international standards and regulations to promote international trade. This requires the evaluation system to be coordinated with the international cosmetic safety evaluation system, reducing trade barriers [3, 6].

2.2 Framework of the cosmetic safety evaluation system

2.2.1 Safety evaluation of raw materials

The safety evaluation of raw materials is the foundation of cosmetic safety evaluation, including the physicochemical properties and toxicological characteristics of raw materials. The safety evaluation of raw materials requires a detailed safety assessment of each raw material used in cosmetics and the risk substances that may be brought in, to ensure that they are harmless to the human body [4, 5, 7].

2.2.2 Safety evaluation of formulations

The safety evaluation of formulations focuses on the overall safety of cosmetic formulations, including the interactions and potential risks among the various components in the formulation. Cosmetic products can generally be considered as combinations of various raw materials and should be assessed based on all raw materials and risk substances. If it is confirmed that there are chemical and/or biological interactions among certain raw materials, the risk substances produced and/or the potential safety risks generated by these interactions should be assessed [8].

2.2.3 Safety evaluation of production processes

The safety evaluation of production processes focuses on the safety issues that may arise during the production process, such as cross-contamination and microbial contamination. The safety evaluation of production processes needs to ensure that the production of cosmetics complies with safety standards to prevent product contamination.

2.2.4 Safety evaluation of products

The safety evaluation of products is the final stage of cosmetic safety evaluation, including the physicochemical stability, microbiological safety, preservative efficacy evaluation, toxicological safety, and compatibility of packaging materials of the products.

2.3 Methods of cosmetic safety evaluation

2.3.1 Laboratory testing

Laboratory testing is the main method of cosmetic safety evaluation, including chemical analysis, microbiological testing, and toxicological testing. Laboratory testing can provide direct evidence of the safety of cosmetics and is an important part of the evaluation system. At present, with the implementation of bans on animal testing for cosmetics in many countries or regions, the development and application of *in vitro* alternative methods and computational toxicology methods are increasingly drawing attention [5, 9].

2.3.2 Clinical trials

Clinical trials are an important means of assessing the safety of cosmetics, evaluating the actual safety of products through human trials. Clinical trials can provide safety data of cosmetics under actual usage conditions, which is crucial for assessing the safety of cosmetics.

2.3.3 Risk assessment

Risk assessment is the core of cosmetic safety evaluation, providing a basis for safety decision-making by assessing the exposure levels and health risks of potential risk substances in cosmetics. The safety assessment of cosmetic products should be exposure-oriented, combining the exposure levels such as the usage method, usage site, usage amount, and residue of the products, to assess the safety of cosmetic products and ensure their safety [2, 5].

2.4 Steps of cosmetic safety risk assessment

2.4.1 Hazard identification

Hazard identification is the first step of risk assessment, that is, based on the results of toxicological tests, clinical research, adverse reaction monitoring, and epidemiological studies of populations, to determine whether there is a potential hazard to human health from the physical, chemical, and toxicological characteristics of raw materials and/or risk substances.

2.4.2 Dose-response relationship assessment

Determine the relationship between the toxicological response of raw materials and/or risk substances and the exposure dose. For threshold toxic effects, the No Observed Adverse Effect Level (NOAEL) or Benchmark Dose (BMD) should be obtained. For non-threshold carcinogenic effects, the dose that causes tumors in 25% of experimental animals (T25) or BMD is used to determine it. For raw materials and/or risk substances with sensitization risks, the No Expected Sensitization Induction Level (NESIL) should also be used to assess their sensitization [6, 8, 10].

2.4.3 Exposure assessment

By assessing the site, concentration, frequency, transdermal absorption rate, and duration of exposure of cosmetic raw materials and/or risk substances to the human body and combining the particularity of the exposed subjects (such as adults, children, infants, etc.), the exposure level is finally determined. When calculating the exposure amount, the possibility of other exposure routes (such as inhalation, ingestion, etc.) should also be considered; if necessary, the exposure situation from other possible sources (such as food and environment, etc.) outside cosmetics should be considered [8].

2.4.4 Risk characterization

It refers to the description of the possibility and degree of damage to human health caused by cosmetic raw materials and/or risk substances. The Margin of Safety (MoS), lifetime cancer risk (LCR), and the comparison between acceptable exposure levels and actual exposure amounts can be used to describe the threshold toxic effects, non-threshold carcinogenic effects, and sensitization effects of cosmetic raw materials and/or risk substances on the human body, respectively [11].

2.5 Challenges and prospects of the cosmetic safety evaluation system

2.5.1 Challenges

The challenges faced by the cosmetic safety evaluation system include the safety evaluation of new raw materials and plant extracts, the application of nanotechnology, and the safety of personalized cosmetics. With the continuous development of the cosmetics industry, new raw materials and technologies are emerging constantly, posing new challenges to the cosmetic safety evaluation system. In addition, since people in different countries or regions have different concepts and habits of cosmetic consumption, there is a significant difference in their systemic exposure to various products. Therefore, it is necessary to carry out real-world investigation and research to supplement the data gap of exposure parameters.

2.5.2 Prospects

The cosmetic safety evaluation system is an important tool for safeguarding consumer health and promoting the development of the cosmetics industry. Through a scientific, comprehensive, dynamic, and internationally coordinated evaluation system, the safety of cosmetics can be effectively assessed, and consumer rights can be protected. In the future, with the progress of science and technology and the changes in consumer demand, the cosmetic safety evaluation system will continue to improve and develop.

2.5.3 Conclusion

Through a scientific, comprehensive, dynamic, and internationally coordinated evaluation system, the safety of cosmetics can be effectively assessed, and consumer rights can be protected. In the future, with the progress of science and technology and the changes in consumer demand, the cosmetic safety evaluation system will continue to improve and develop.

3. Construction of an evidence-based system for cosmetic efficacy evaluation

The establishment of an evidence-based system for cosmetic efficacy evaluation is a complex and systematic project that requires scientific and rigorous design from multiple key dimensions. First and foremost, it is of utmost importance to deeply explore the internal mechanisms by which different functions exert their effects. For instance, the whitening effect may involve multiple mechanisms such as inhibiting the activity of tyrosinase and hindering the production and transportation of melanin. On the other hand, the anti-wrinkle effect may be closely related to promoting collagen synthesis and enhancing the metabolism of skin cells. Only by accurately understanding these mechanisms can a solid theoretical foundation be provided for subsequent efficacy evaluations. Secondly, the rational selection of efficacy markers directly impacts the accuracy and reliability of the evaluation results. Markers should be specific and capable of precisely reflecting the claimed functions of cosmetics. For example, for the moisturizing effect, the water content of the skin stratum corneum can be selected as a key marker. In the case of the antioxidant effect, the level of intracellular reactive oxygen species (ROS) may be a more appropriate marker. Furthermore, experimental design is the core part of the entire evidence-based system. Basic principles such as randomization, control, and replication should be adhered to ensure the scientific nature and reproducibility of experimental results. When designing an experimental plan, numerous factors need to be comprehensively considered, including sample size, grouping methods, intervention measures, observation indicators, and time points. In addition, every detail in the testing process cannot be overlooked. The screening of subjects should strictly follow established standards to ensure their representativeness and to exclude interfering factors. For example, for the evaluation of anti-aging effects, subjects whose age and skin type meet specific conditions should be selected to avoid excessive individual differences from affecting the experimental results. Testers need to receive professional and systematic training, master various testing techniques and methods proficiently, and ensure the accuracy and consistency of operations. At the same time, the correct operation of testing equipment is also crucial for ensuring data quality. Equipment should be calibrated and maintained regularly to ensure its stable performance. Moreover, external conditions such as environmental temperature and humidity may also affect the testing results. Therefore, the experimental environment needs to be strictly controlled and maintained within an appropriate temperature and humidity range, and the interference of environmental factors on the experiment should be minimized. Next, I will elaborate on some efficacy categories about which consumers are more concerned.

3.1 Construction of an evidence-based system for evaluating the efficacy of cosmetics related to skin anti: Aging

3.1.1 Overview of skin aging

Aging is defined as a time-dependent, ongoing change in the functionality and reproduction of higher organisms, associated with a greater likelihood of morbidity and mortality [12]. Skin aging is a complex biological process marked by various physiological changes that occur over time, in which human skin is continually subjected to both intrinsic and extrinsic factors that affect its functionality as it ages [13]. A comprehensive understanding of the hallmarks of skin aging is essential for the formulation of effective skincare interventions. Rigorous evaluation of the efficacy of skincare products is critical to ensure they effectively mitigate the signs of aging and enhance skin health, ultimately supporting individuals in maintaining a youthful appearance and improving their self-esteem.

Recently, study has outlined seven hallmarks related to skin aging: (1) genomic instability (DNA damage) and telomere attrition; (2) epigenetic alterations and loss of proteostasis; (3) deregulated skin nutrient-sensing; (4) mitochondrial dysfunction; (5) cellular senescence in skin; (6) stem cell exhaustion and dysregulation; and (7) altered intracellular communication (**Figure 1**) [14]. The first two hallmarks are recognized as primary hallmarks in that they attribute to the skin damage that initiates the aging process. The third to the fifth hallmarks are categorized as antagonistic hallmarks in that they are the responses to damage that attempt to counteract the effects of aging. The last two hallmarks are integrative hallmarks that are the factors contributing to the observable characteristics and phenotypes of aging skin [3]. Each of these hallmarks can be interconnected with one another during the process of skin aging, contributing to the aging phenotype.

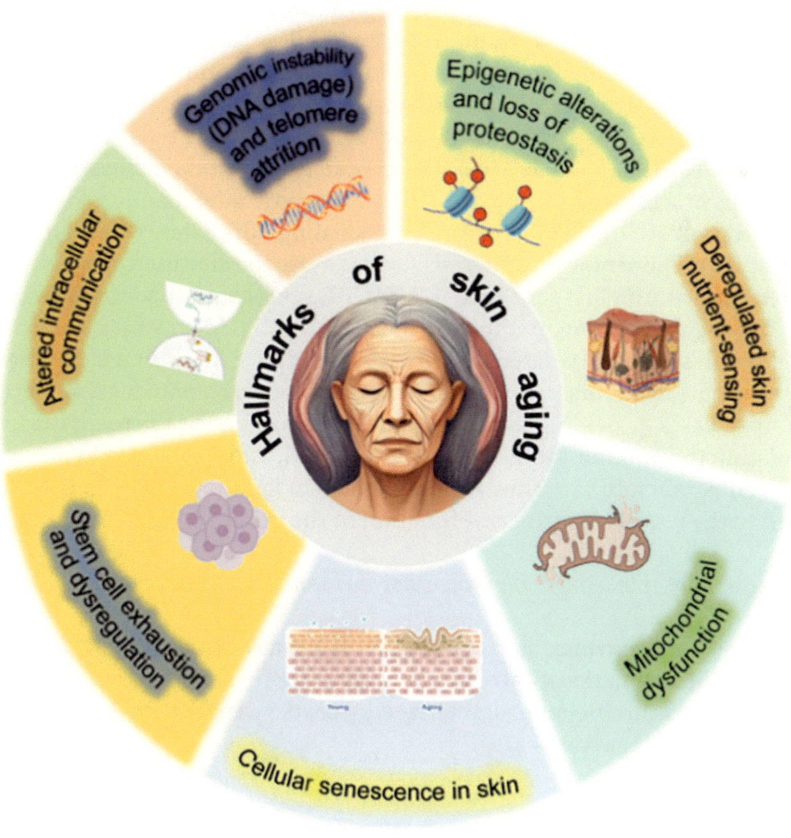

Figure 1.
Hallmarks of skin aging.

3.1.2 Mechanisms of skin aging

Intrinsic skin aging refers to the natural aging process of the skin that occurs due to time, genetic factors, and biological changes within the body, leading to a natural decline in collagen and elastin production, reduced cell turnover, and decreased barrier functions [15]. For example, there is a simultaneous decline in both the number and functionality of fibroblasts, resulting in both the quantity and thickness of collagen fibers to diminish and leading to a higher ratio of type III collagen compared to type I collagen [16]. Aged skin also exhibits fragmentation of dermal collagen and elastin, resulting in reduced skin elasticity and firmness [17]. Additionally, the proliferation rate of the cell in basal layer declines, resulting in thinning in both epidermis and epidermal–dermal junction [13].

Extrinsic skin aging refers to the accelerated aging of the skin caused by environmental factors such as air pollution, solar radiation, smoking, and nutrition [18]. Notably, photoaging due to ultraviolet (UV) radiation is the most significant contributor to extrinsic skin aging. UVA (320–400 nm) and UVB (280–320 nm) rays reach the earth in considerable amounts, posing risks to skin structures by directly inducing DNA damage and indirectly causing genetic instability through the generation of reactive oxygen species (ROS). UVB radiation primarily induces cyclobutane dimers (CPDs), while 8-hydroxy-2-deoxyguanine (8-OHdG) is a common marker for assessing DNA damage from UVA exposure [19]. Furthermore, ROS elicited by UV rays activate nuclear factor kappa-B (NF-kB), leading to increased expression of pro-inflammatory cytokines such as IL-1α, IL-6, and TNF-α [20], contributing to inflammatory disorders. Additionally, exposure to infrared radiation (IR; 760 nm–1 mm) has harmful effects, including the induction of matrix metalloproteinase (MMP) expression, collagen degradation, and an increase in skin mast cells [21].

Indeed, both intrinsic and extrinsic factors can lead to irreversible senescence in skin cells. This process is driven by telomere shortening, mitochondrial dysfunction, and the activation of DNA damage response signaling, ultimately resulting in cell cycle arrest [13]. The senescent skin cells demonstrate the elevation age-associated biomarkers such as p16INK4a, p21Waf-1, HMGB1, senescence-associated beta-galactosidase (SA-β-gal), and downregulation in lamin B1 [22]. Meanwhile, senescent cells also exhibit senescence-associated secretory phenotype (SASP), in which they induce altered secretome including pro-inflammatory cytokines, chemokines, and growth factors or proteases, providing influential consequences on the microenvironment by modulating the immune system, remodeling ECM, and altering cellular functions [23]. Altogether, the accumulation of senescent keratinocytes and fibroblasts is attributed to the loss of integrity and function of the skin.

3.1.3 Visible signs of skin aging with underlying mechanisms

The intrinsic and extrinsic skin aging differ in terms of their clinical traits and visible signs. The hallmarks of intrinsic skin aging are fine lines, laxity, and xerosis, whereas extrinsic skin aging is characterized by coarse wrinkles, irregular pigmentation, and lentigines (age spots) [18].

3.1.3.1 Fine lines and laxity

Fine lines and skin laxity are both indicators of aging caused by intrinsic and extrinsic factors impacting the skin. Fine lines are defined as small, shallow creases that develop primarily due to the thinning of the epidermis and a reduction in collagen and elastin levels. In contrast, skin laxity refers to the skin's diminished ability to regain its original shape after being stretched, resulting in a loose and sagging appearance due to a loss of firmness and elasticity.

The development of fine lines and laxity is primarily driven by age-related degradation of collagen, elastin, chondroitin, and hyaluronic acid in fibroblasts. This process is accompanied by an increased expression of matrix metalloproteinases (MMPs), which are enzymes that break down components of the extracellular matrix (ECM) [24]. Together, these changes contribute to the visible signs of aging in the skin. Meanwhile, the intrinsic aging-related generation of ROS also contributes to these processes [25]. Other age-related factors like hormonal change, weight loss, or gravity also contribute to skin contour deformities [26]. Nevertheless, the induction of these fine wrinkles can be different among diverse ethnical groups with varied anatomical regions [27].

3.1.3.2 Xerosis (skin dryness)

Dry skin, or xerosis, is a common dermatological condition affected by various factors, including hydration levels, sebum production, and environmental influences. The condition is often linked to an age-associated alteration in skin barrier function, particularly in the stratum corneum [28]. As skin ages, there is a notable reduction in both the size and secretory activity of sebocytes, leading to a significant decline in surface lipids and skin hydration [25]. Indeed, in menopausal women, research indicates a marked increase in the pH of the hydro-lipid film and a reduction in sebum production. Moreover, the expression of osmolyte transporters such as SMIT and TAUT is also negatively correlated with age, which further affected water homeostasis by decreasing the keratinocyte volume and leading to xerosis [29].

3.1.3.3 Coarse wrinkles

Coarse wrinkles are deep lines with a rough texture that appear on the skin. Compared to intrinsic skin aging, the extrinsically induced tissue damage is more pronounced in the epidermis and dermis. Chronic UV exposure over extended periods significantly disrupts the normal skin architecture, with many histological changes associated, with photoaging being the most evident in the ECM of the dermis [30]. Notably, the dermal elastic fibers are profoundly affected by UV radiation. In response to photodamage and photoaging, ROS accumulation further induced the damage of DNA, proteins, and lipids, which affects the skin-repair function [25]. Moreover, upon UV exposure, elastic fibers initially undergo hyperplastic changes, leading to an increase in the amount of elastic tissue produced [31].

3.1.3.4 Lentigines (age spots)

Age spots, or lentigines, are hyperpigmented macules resulting from increased melanocyte proliferation that associate with age, chronic sun exposure, or other exposome like air pollution [32]. Recent study also discovered that chronic inflammation and the infiltration of pro-inflammatory M1 macrophages also contributed to lentigines formation [33]. The occurrence of lentigines is marked by changes throughout the entire skin structure, including the epidermis, the dermal-epidermal junction, and the dermis [34]. The formation of lentigines is attributed to the accumulation of photoaged cells, which are characterized by the presence of lipofuscin bodies and changed keratinocyte proliferation [26]. Furthermore, the formation of rete ridges in the affected epidermis impedes the upward migration of melanin in the basal layer [35]. Concurrently, a deficiency in SDF1 serves as a significant stimulus for melanogenic processes, exacerbating the mottled pigmentation characteristic of age spots [36].

3.1.4 Evaluation methods for skin aging

3.1.4.1 Cell-based in vitro method

In vitro methods for evaluating skin aging use cell models that simulate the human physiological environment. Advances in cell culture technology are shifting from 2D to co-cultures and 3D skin models, enabling better assessments of raw materials and cosmetics.

2D monolayer cell cultures involve the application of human keratinocytes and fibroblasts. Commonly used human skin fibroblasts include HFF-1 (Human Foreskin Fibroblasts), BJ (Bjerknes Fibroblasts), and HDF (Human Dermal Fibroblasts), whereas epidermal keratinocyte cell lines frequently used in research are HaCaT and NHEK (Normal Human Epidermal Keratinocytes). Researchers often use hydrogen peroxide (H_2O_2) or UV stress to model extrinsic skin aging, while intrinsic aging models are less common [37]. Since UVB affects the epidermis and UVA penetrates the dermis, models expose HDF/HFF-1 cells to UVB and NHEK/HaCaT cells to UVA. In addition to fibroblasts and keratinocytes, melanocytes are also used in studies of skin aging. For example, NHEM (Normal Human Epidermal Melanocytes) is utilized to understand the processes associated with skin aging [38].

In terms of 3D culture models, these are advanced *in vitro* constructs that replicate the structure and function of human skin. Commercially available reconstructed skin models include EpiDerm™, SkinEthic™, and Episkin™ currently widely used in studying skin aging [39]. Moreover, bio-printed models incorporate skin cells such as keratinocytes, fibroblasts, and melanocytes, which are also able to create human skin equivalents [40]. Other than these, skin organoid cultures and "skin-on-chip" technologies also provide detailed representation of skin in vivo, allowing the study of intricate tissue interactions during aging [41].

The most common experiments for assessing anti-aging activities focus on various effects. Cell proliferation and viability tests typically employ CCK8 (Cell Counting Kit-8) or MTT (3-(4,5-Dimethylthiazol-2-yl)-2,5-Diphenyltetrazolium Bromide) assays. Antioxidation experiments assess oxidative stress-related factors such as superoxide dismutase (SOD), malondialdehyde (MDA), reduced glutathione (GSH), catalase (CAT), and reactive oxygen species (ROS) [42]. Additionally, collagen production and matrix metalloproteinase (MMP) assays are widely used in cellular skin aging studies [37]. The expression levels of hyaluronan synthases (HAS1, HAS2, and HAS3), which are involved in hyaluronic acid synthesis, are commonly used as age-related markers for skin moisture [43]. Other senescence-related biomarkers found in skin tissues, directly linked to senescence hallmarks, are listed in the table below (**Table 1**) [22]. Each of these assays has unique features, and typical techniques such as immunoassay (ELISA), RT-qPCR, flow cytometry, immunofluorescence, and Western blotting can be employed for identification.

Marker	Gene name	Related skin aging hallmark	Identification methods
CDKN2A ($p16^{INK4A}$)	Cyclin-dependent kinase inhibitor 2A	cellular senescence	immunoblot, RT–qPCR, WB, IHC, IF, FISH, immunostaining
CDKN1A ($p21^{CIP1}$)	Cyclin-dependent kinase inhibitor 1A	cellular senescence	immunoblot, RT–qPCR, WB, IHC, IF
IL-6	Interleukin-6	SASP	Immunoblot, RT–qPCR, WB, microarray, immunoassay (ELISA), IF, IHC
TNF	Tumor necrosis factor	SASP	Immunoblot, RT–qPCR, WB, microarray, immunoassay (ELISA), IF, IHC
H2AX	H2A.X variant histone	genomic instability	IF, IHC, WB, RT–qPCR
IL-1α	Interleukin-1α	SASP	RT–qPCR, immunoassay (ELISA), flow cytometry
IL-1β	Interleukin-1β	SASP	RT–qPCR, microarray, WB, cytokine array, immunoassay (ELISA), IHC, IF
SA-β-gal	Senescence-associated β-galactosidase	cellular senescence	Colorimetric and fluorescent staining and microscopy, IHC, IF, X-Gal crystal detection via electron microscopy, flow cytometry, SA-β-gal staining, X-gal precipitation
CXCL8	C–X–C motif chemokine ligand 8	SASP	Immunoassay (ELISA), RT–qPCR
HMGB1	High-mobility group box 1	genomic instability	RT–qPCR, IHC, IF, WB, ELISA
MMP2	Matrix metallopeptidase 2	SASP	WB, immunoassay (ELISA), RT–qPCR, IHC
CXCL10	HGNC:10637	SASP	immunoassay (ELISA), RT–qPCR, flow cytometry
MMP3	Matrix metallopeptidase 3	SASP	RT–qPCR, immunoassay, microarray, ELISA, IHC
MMP9	Matrix metallopeptidase 9	SASP	RT–qPCR, immunoassay (ELISA)
LMNB1	Lamin B1	cellular senescence	IF, RT–qPCR, WB
MMP1	Matrix metallopeptidase 1	SASP	immunoassay (ELISA), RT–qPCR
Telomere length	Telomere length	telomere attrition	FISH, TRAP assay, RT–qPCR
Lipofuscin	Lipofuscin	cellular senescence	Sudan Black B staining
MKI67	Marker of proliferation Ki-67	cellular senescence	IF

Marker	Gene name	Related skin aging hallmark	Identification methods
TAF	Telomere-associated foci	telomere attrition	ImmunoFISH
TP53BP1	Tumor protein p53 binding protein 1	genomic instability	IF, IHC, IF foci

Table 1.
Senescence-related markers in skin.

3.1.4.2 Human efficacy evaluation

3.1.4.2.1 Methods for testing skin firmness and hydration

As skin ages, its hydration, elasticity, and overall biomechanical properties change significantly. Several advanced techniques are employed to assess these factors, providing insights into skin condition.

Corneometry with suction method is a technique that uses negative pressure to draw skin into a test probe equipped with optical systems for measuring skin displacement over time. Common corneometer, like the MPA580-Cutometer, evaluates the hydration of the outer layer of the stratum corneum [44]. The water content in the stratum corneum affects the capacitor's behavior, resulting in changes in its capacity that correspond to the skin's hydration levels [45]. Another instrument includes the Frictiometer ® FR700, which measures skin friction. It operates by rotating a Teflon cylindrical probe; a smoother skin results in lower torque and friction values, while dry, wrinkled skin exhibits higher friction.

Pressure method is based on Young's modulus, which describes the material's resistance to deformation under stress. The Skin Elastimeter is a compact, portable instrument used to assess skin elasticity through indentometry. It features a central tip on a reference plate, and when applied to the skin, it causes a temporary indentation of up to 0.3 mm. A built-in sensor measures the force needed to create this indentation, allowing for the calculation of the skin's immediate elasticity [46]. Instruments like the Delfin ElastiMeter utilize this principle to assess skin elasticity. Another method includes the torsion method, in which a central disk is adhered to the skin, with a ring attached to it. By applying torque, the angle of rotation is measured to evaluate skin elasticity [47]. The Dia-stron Dermal Torque Meter DTM is a representative device for this method.

Transepidermal water loss (TEWL) is a crucial indicator of skin barrier function and hydration levels. The Tewameter® TM 300 is a non-invasive device specifically designed to measure TEWL. It features a probe with a sensitive sensor that is applied to the skin's surface to assess water evaporation over time. By detecting the rate of water vapor loss, it provides valuable insights into the integrity of the skin's barrier.

Shear Wave Propagation assesses skin viscoelasticity by analyzing the acoustic waves in the frequency of 0.5-30 kHz [48]. Other devices, such as the BCT2000 for measuring biomechanical properties, the Venustron for soft tissue testing, the Extensometer for stretch testing, and the BLS700 Ballistometer for impact testing, also provide scientific evidence for claims of skin firmness.

3.1.4.2.2 Methods for testing skin roughness and anti-wrinkle efficacy

Dry, rough skin with wrinkles is a characteristic of aging. Key parameters for assessing skin roughness include friction, roughness, and smoothness. Anti-wrinkle efficacy refers to the ability to reduce the appearance of wrinkles or make them less noticeable. Changes in various physical and chemical indicators, such as the number, length, volume, area, and depth of wrinkles, are important metrics for assessing skin aging. Common methods include 3D imaging analysis, 2D image analysis, and profilometry.

The use of 3D skin imaging systems combined with computer image processing is a standard method for evaluating wrinkle parameters due to its speed, accuracy, and high resolution. Instruments like the Primos® system and the EvaSKIN and EvaFACE systems (which focus on localized and full-face assessments, respectively) examine alterations in skin structure by evaluating isotropy parameters [49].

Portable 3D imaging systems like the C-Cube from Pixience and Antera 3D from MIRAVEX enable rapid and precise assessment of skin texture and wrinkles. These devices utilize computer-assisted surface reconstruction and multidirectional lighting to enhance user engagement and provide clear image analysis [50].

Devices like the VISIA or VISIA-CR facial analysis systems capture images under standard, UV, or polarized light [51]. Specialized software like Mirror Photo Tools and Image-Pro Plus can analyze these images for relevant wrinkle parameters. Profilometry methods, including laser, optical, and mechanical skin profiling, also enable quantitative wrinkle analysis. Instruments like the Visioline® VL650 utilize these techniques, often requiring silicone replicas of the skin surface for accurate assessments to assess skin macro-relief parameters [52].

The VisioScan ® VC20 plus system uses a uniform UV light source and a high-resolution CCD camera to capture images of the skin's surface. The SELS software analyzes the grayscale distribution, providing clinically relevant parameters: skin smoothness (SEsm), roughness (SEr), desquamation level (SEsc), and wrinkle status (SEw). This high-resolution UV imaging method offers a simple, cost-effective, and accurate approach for evaluating cosmetic efficacy by directly assessing skin surface morphology and dryness.

3.1.4.2.3 Methods for testing skin structure

Aging affects the physiological structure of the skin. Device like the Ultrascan UC22 utilizes a 22 MHz ultrasound frequency to produce high-resolution images of skin at depths of 8–10 mm, allowing analysis of skin thickness, cross-sectional area, and aging severity. Similarly, the high-frequency ultrasound probes from DermaLab Combo® by Cortex and DermaScan C can conduct related tests. Other devices like the Two-Photon Excitation Microscopy (TPEM) and MPT flex (Multiphoton Tomography) employ near-infrared femtosecond laser technology for sub-micron spatial resolution in skin optical biopsy, allowing visualization of dermal collagen and elastin fibers *in vivo* and making them suitable for studying skin aging [53].

Line-field confocal optical coherence tomography (LC-OCT) is another type of non-invasive imaging technique that merges the principles of optical coherence tomography and reflectance confocal microscopy with line-field illumination [54]. It produces cell-resolved images of the skin in various orientations, including vertical, horizontal, and three-dimensional views. Since LC-OCT generates substantial data, automated deep learning algorithms are highly relevant for aiding image analysis.

The LC-OCT also covers algorithms designed for skin layer segmentation and keratinocyte nuclei segmentation.

3.2 Evaluation of cosmetics products for sensitive skin: Methods and approaches

Sensitive skin has become a significant concern in both dermatology and the cosmetic industry, with more consumers seeking products that are gentle yet effective. However, the evaluation of cosmetic products for sensitive skin is a complex task, as sensitive skin reacts differently to various stimuli compared to normal skin types. Determining whether a cosmetic product is suitable for sensitive skin requires a combination of subjective assessments, objective measurements, and clinical testing. This essay will explore the methods used to evaluate the suitability of cosmetics for sensitive skin, focusing on product safety, effectiveness, and consumer experience.

3.2.1 Overview of sensitive skin

Sensitive skin refers to a skin type that exhibits heightened reactions to environmental factors, skincare products, or internal triggers, such as stress or hormonal changes. People with sensitive skin often experience symptoms such as redness, irritation, itching, or burning sensations when exposed to stimuli that do not affect individuals with normal skin. These reactions are often linked to a compromised skin barrier, which makes the skin more prone to irritation and allergic reactions.

The evaluation of cosmetic products suitable for sensitive skin is essential for ensuring both the safety and efficacy of products designed to soothe or avoid triggering sensitive skin reactions. Cosmetic products, including moisturizers, cleansers, sunscreens, and makeup, need to be evaluated to ensure that they do not exacerbate skin issues like irritation, dryness, or redness.

3.2.1.1 Purpose of evaluation methods

The primary objectives of evaluating cosmetic products for sensitive skin are:

- *To ensure product safety*: This includes determining that a product does not cause irritation, allergic reactions, or any other adverse effects on sensitive skin.

- *To assess product effectiveness*: Evaluating how well the product can soothe or enhance the condition of sensitive skin, such as improving hydration, reducing irritation, and strengthening the skin barrier.

Cosmetic products are typically evaluated using both subjective methods (such as consumer surveys and expert assessments) and objective measurements (such as skin hydration and barrier function tests). Combining these methods ensures that the products meet both safety and performance standards.

3.2.2 Challenges in evaluating cosmetics for sensitive skin

3.2.2.1 Variability in individual skin sensitivity

One of the major challenges in evaluating cosmetics for sensitive skin is the variability of individual skin responses. Sensitive skin is not a uniform condition, and different people may react to the same product in different ways. Factors such as age, genetics, skin type, and lifestyle can all influence how an individual's skin responds to a particular cosmetic product. This variability makes it difficult to establish universal standards for evaluating cosmetic products.

3.2.2.2 Subjective nature of consumer experiences

While clinical testing can provide objective data, the subjective experiences of consumers play a significant role in determining whether a product is truly suitable for sensitive skin. Many people with sensitive skin rely on their own experiences, such as sensations of stinging, burning, or itching, to gauge whether a product is suitable for them. This makes it essential to include consumer feedback and self-reported assessments in product evaluation.

3.2.2.3 Environmental and lifestyle factors

Skin sensitivity can also be influenced by external factors such as temperature, humidity, pollution, and the use of other skincare products. For instance, harsh weather conditions or the use of certain makeup products can exacerbate skin sensitivity. Thus, evaluating cosmetics for sensitive skin requires consideration of these factors to assess how the product interacts with the skin in real-world conditions.

3.2.3 Evaluation methods for cosmetics products

3.2.3.1 Subjective assessment methods

3.2.3.1.1 Self-reported questionnaires

Self-reported questionnaires are commonly used to gather insights from consumers about their experiences with cosmetic products. These questionnaires ask participants to assess the product's effects on their skin, including any symptoms like irritation, redness, or discomfort.

To evaluate cosmetics products for sensitive skin, self-reported questionnaires could be collected pre- and post-cosmetics product usage.

- *Examples of questionnaires*:
    - Sensitive Skin Questionnaire (SSQ) [55, 56]: This tool helps assess the degree of skin sensitivity based on responses to environmental stimuli and product use.
    - Dermatological Life Quality Index (DLQI) [57, 58]: This tool evaluates how skin conditions (like sensitivity) impact a person's daily life, focusing on physical and emotional well-being.
- *Benefits*: Self-reported questionnaires provide valuable information about how products perform in real-world conditions and offer insights into consumer satisfaction.
- *Limitations*: The subjective nature of self-reporting means results can vary based on individual perceptions, experiences, and expectations.

3.2.3.1.2 Interviews and consumer feedback

In-depth interviews or focus groups can provide a more detailed understanding of how consumers perceive a product's impact on their sensitive skin. These methods can help identify specific irritants or beneficial effects that might not be captured in standardized questionnaires.

- *Importance*: Detailed interviews allow for exploring how specific ingredients or formulations interact with sensitive skin, providing insights that may not be immediately apparent through clinical testing.

3.2.3.2 Objective assessment methods

3.2.3.2.1 Patch testing

Patch testing is a well-established method used to determine if a cosmetic product causes skin irritation or allergic reactions. In this test, small quantities of a product are applied to patches of skin (usually on the back or inner arm) and left for a specified time (typically 48–72 hours). The area is then observed for signs of redness, swelling, or blistering [59].

- *Use in sensitive skin*: Patch testing helps identify whether a product triggers irritation or allergic responses in sensitive skin, such as rashes or eczema-like symptoms.

3.2.3.2.2 TEWL (transepidermal water loss) measurement

TEWL is a critical measure of skin barrier function and is especially useful in assessing products designed for sensitive skin. Increased TEWL is indicative of a compromised barrier, which is common in sensitive skin [60, 61].

- *Procedure*: A specialized device, such as a Tewameter®, measures the amount of water lost through the skin's surface.
- *Use in sensitive skin*: Products that help restore barrier integrity and reduce TEWL are considered beneficial for sensitive skin.

3.2.3.2.3 Clinical irritation testing

This test involves applying a product to a controlled area of the skin and monitoring it for any signs of irritation, redness, or other adverse effects. Irritation testing can be conducted in a clinical setting to assess how a product behaves under typical conditions of sensitive skin [62, 63].

- *Use in sensitive skin*: Clinical irritation testing helps determine if a product is too harsh for sensitive skin or if it provides a soothing effect without causing adverse reactions.

3.2.3.2.4 Skin hydration and barrier function assessments

In addition to TEWL, skin hydration levels are a key indicator of skin health. Sensitive skin often exhibits reduced hydration due to a weakened barrier function [64].

- *Method*: Corneometry is often used to measure skin hydration levels. A well-hydrated skin barrier is essential for reducing irritation and sensitivity. Cosmetics that improve hydration and strengthen the skin's barrier are highly beneficial [65].

3.2.3.2.5 Facial stinging test

The facial stinging test [66], particularly the lactic acid sting test (LAST), is a widely used method to evaluate the reactivity of sensitive skin. It specifically measures subjective sensations of discomfort, such as stinging, burning, or tingling, after applying a potential irritant to the face. Here's a detailed look at this test.

3.2.3.2.5.1 Procedure

- *Participant selection*:
    - Test subjects are typically chosen based on self-reported sensitivity or dermatologist assessment.
    - Subjects often have a history of sensitive skin but no active dermatological conditions (e.g., eczema, rosacea) during testing.
- *Test substance*:
    - Commonly used substances include lactic acid (5–10%), a known irritant for sensitive skin.
    - The cosmetic product being tested can also be directly applied.
- *Application*:
    - Commonly used substances include lactic acid (5–10%), a known irritant for sensitive skin.
    - The cosmetic product being tested can also be directly applied.
- *Observation period*:
    - The subject is asked to report any sensations of stinging, burning, or discomfort over a set time, typically 2–10 minutes.
- *Scoring*:
    - Reactions are rated on a subjective scale (e.g., 0 = no stinging, 1 = mild, 2 = moderate, 3 = severe).
    - Some protocols also record visible signs of irritation, though the test primarily focuses on subjective sensations.

3.2.3.2.6 Forearm tape stripping and capsaicin application test

Forearm Tape Stripping and Capsaicin Application Test (FA-TS-CAT) was developed as an alternative to traditional facial stinging tests for sensitive skin evaluation [65].

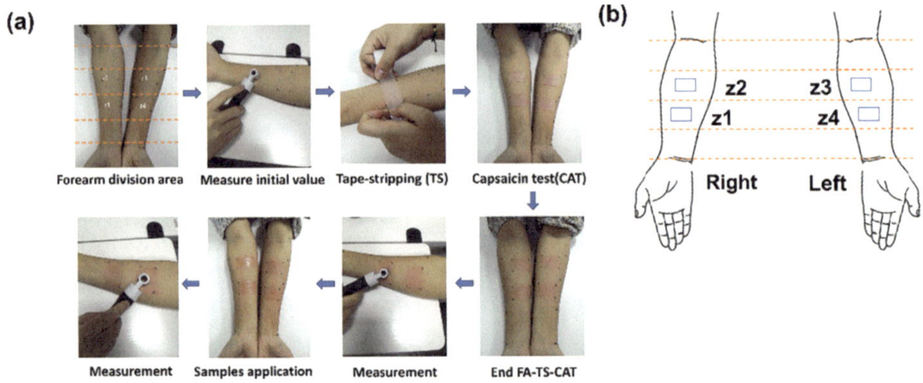

It combines tape stripping (to mimic facial skin sensitivity) and capsaicin application (to induce irritation), which accurately simulates the natural recovery trend observed in sensitive skin following product application. This model not only enhances assessment efficiency but also ensures higher safety and adherence of subjects, providing a practical tool for the development and validation of sensitive skincare products and treatments.

3.2.3.2.6.1 Procedure

1. Preparation

   - *Participant selection*:

     - o Participants with varying degrees of skin sensitivity are chosen, often including both sensitive and normal skin types for comparison.

   - *Site selection*:

     - o The volar forearm is typically used due to its accessibility and relatively uniform skin properties.

2. Tape Stripping (TS)

   - *Purpose*: To partially disrupt the skin barrier by removing layers of the stratum corneum.

   - *Process*:

     - o Adhesive tape is repeatedly applied and removed from a specific area of the forearm.

     - o The number of strips (usually 10–15) is standardized to achieve controlled disruption.

     - o The degree of disruption can be measured using transepidermal water loss (TEWL).

DOI: http://dx.doi.org/10.5772/intechopen.1009010

3. Capsaicin Application (CAT)

    - *Purpose*: To test the sensory response of the skin. Capsaicin, the active component in chili peppers, stimulates nociceptors (pain-sensitive nerve endings).

    - *Process*:

        - A small amount of capsaicin solution (e.g., 0.01%–0.1%) is applied to the stripped area.

        - Capsaicin is left on the skin for a fixed duration, typically a few minutes.

4. Observation and scoring

    - *Sensory response*: Participants report sensations such as burning, stinging, or tingling using a standardized scale (e.g., 0 = no sensation, 10 = unbearable).

    - *Visual assessment*: Redness, swelling, or other visible signs of irritation are recorded.

5. Post-test evaluation

    - *Recovery monitoring*: TEWL or other skin recovery parameters may be measured over time to assess how quickly the barrier function is restored.

3.2.4 Clinical trials and controlled studies with sensitive skin subjects

Clinical trials play a central role in evaluating the safety and effectiveness of cosmetic products for sensitive skin. These trials typically involve randomized controlled studies (RCTs) where participants are either given the product or a placebo, and their skin's response is carefully monitored over time. The demand for products formulated specifically for sensitive skin increases, and there is a growing emphasis on scientifically sound evaluation methods. These methods aim to ensure that cosmetics are not only effective but also safe for individuals with sensitive skin, who are more prone to reactions such as irritation, itching, and redness. Evaluating the suitability of cosmetic products for sensitive skin involves both subjective and objective testing techniques to assess the product's safety, performance, and long-term benefits.

3.2.5 Technological advances in cosmetics evaluation

With the rapid development of technology, new tools and techniques have emerged to enhance the evaluation process. These advances enable more accurate and comprehensive assessments of how cosmetic products interact with sensitive skin, providing both consumers and manufacturers with valuable insights.

3.2.5.1 Role of artificial intelligence (AI) in skin evaluation

Artificial intelligence (AI) has been increasingly integrated into dermatological and cosmetic research, offering new ways to analyze skin data and predict how products will perform on sensitive skin. AI can be applied to various aspects of skin evaluation:

3.2.6 Discussion

The evaluation of cosmetics for sensitive skin is a multifaceted process that requires both subjective and objective testing methods to ensure that products are safe, effective, and beneficial for individuals with skin sensitivity. With advancements in technology and clinical testing, the industry is continually improving its ability to cater to sensitive skin concerns.

As the demand for sensitive skin solutions grows, future developments will likely include even more personalized skincare options, aided by AI and wearable technology, to offer real-time assessments of how products interact with individual skin types. Ensuring safety and efficacy will remain paramount, and as consumer awareness increases, more sophisticated testing and reporting methods will drive the development of better products tailored to the needs of sensitive skin.

3.3 Leveraging artificial intelligence for evidence-based cosmetic evaluation: Safety, efficacy, and mildness

Artificial intelligence (AI) is revolutionizing multiple industries, and the cosmetic sector is no exception [67–69]. In the context of evaluating the safety, efficacy, and mildness of cosmetic products, AI presents an opportunity to enhance and accelerate traditional evaluation methods. By utilizing AI-driven tools, the cosmetic industry can better predict risks, analyze large datasets, optimize formulations, and ultimately deliver products that meet consumer demands for safety, efficacy, and mildness with greater precision [67]. In this section, we explore how AI technologies can be integrated into evidence-based cosmetic evaluation systems, providing more accurate and timely results, reducing reliance on animal testing, and improving overall product development.

3.3.1 AI in safety evaluation: Predicting toxicity and irritation risks

Traditionally, the safety of cosmetic products has been evaluated through *in vivo* (animal) and *in vitro* (cell culture) testing, which can be time-consuming, expensive, and ethically challenging. AI, particularly machine learning (ML) algorithms, has the potential to dramatically enhance safety evaluations by predicting toxicity and irritation risks based on chemical structures, ingredient interactions, and biological response models [70].

3.3.1.1 Predictive toxicology

Molecular Modeling and Virtual Screening: One of the primary ways AI contributes to safety evaluation is through predictive toxicology. Machine learning models can analyze chemical structures and predict their potential toxicity [60, 61]. Trained on extensive datasets such as the Toxicology Data Network (TOXNET) and EPA databases, these AI systems can identify patterns between molecular features and toxicological outcomes. This enables the prediction of how new cosmetic ingredients might behave in human systems, reducing the need for animal testing. Recent advances in deep learning (DL) allow for more accurate predictions, even with complex molecular interactions [71, 72]. These models can also help identify previously overlooked toxicological concerns, ensuring products meet safety standards without unnecessary experimentation.

In Silico Models for Dermal Absorption: Another promising application is the prediction of dermal absorption and skin irritation. AI models simulate how cosmetic ingredients penetrate the skin barrier and predict potential irritation or allergic reactions. This process, enhanced by datasets from *in vitro* tests and clinical studies, could significantly reduce human and animal testing. AI-powered simulations help create more realistic models of skin responses, leading to more accurate safety evaluations [72].

3.3.1.2 Risk assessment models

Quantitative Structure-Activity Relationship (QSAR) Models: AI-powered QSAR models evaluate ingredient toxicity by correlating chemical structure with biological activity. These models use databases of known substances to predict hazards for novel ingredients by comparing their chemical structures with those of known toxic or non-toxic compounds. The growing use of AI in QSAR models helps cosmetic companies avoid harmful substances and enhance the safety of new formulations [67, 71, 72].

Adverse Outcome Pathways (AOP): AI can also be employed to map adverse outcome pathways (AOPs), which describe the sequence of biological events from chemical exposure to adverse health effects [72]. AI tools aggregate data from various sources to build comprehensive AOP networks, improving understanding of how specific ingredients might cause skin damage, allergic reactions, or systemic toxicity. This approach is increasingly important for refining ingredient safety assessments, ensuring that cosmetic formulations are both effective and safe.

3.3.2 AI in efficacy evaluation: Enhancing clinical trials and consumer insights

While safety is a critical concern, the efficacy of cosmetic products is equally important. AI can streamline and enhance efficacy evaluation by improving clinical trial design, analyzing consumer feedback, and simulating real-world usage scenarios to predict product performance [67, 73–75].

3.3.2.1 Optimizing clinical trials and operations

Predicting Efficacy in Different Skin Types: AI can help predict how individuals with varying skin types or conditions (e.g., dry skin, acne-prone skin) will respond to cosmetic products [67]. By analyzing data from previous clinical trials, dermatological studies, and skin physiology databases, AI can segment consumers into more accurate subgroups. This targeted approach ensures that clinical trials are more reflective of real-world usage, improving the relevance and efficiency of product evaluations [67, 73].

Simulating Long-Term Efficacy: Long-term efficacy testing, particularly for products targeting aging, skin elasticity, or hydration, often requires extensive trials. AI models can simulate the long-term effects of cosmetic products, predicting their impact over months or years without the need for prolonged human trials. This significantly reduces the cost and time associated with clinical testing, accelerating product development while ensuring reliability in efficacy predictions [67, 73].

Minimal Clinical Trials and Precise Operation: Over the past decade, esthetic dermatology has seen major innovations to treat various skin issues, such as acne scars, pigmentation, skin aging, and blood vessel problems. However, many esthetic treatments still carry risks, especially for patients with different skin types or complex sensitive skin conditions. The advent of AI presents a promising solution, offering greater precision, safety, and personalized care for these treatments [74, 75].

3.3.2.2 Consumer data analysis

AI tools can analyze vast amounts of consumer feedback from social media, product reviews, and forums. Natural language processing (NLP) algorithms can mine text data to identify common sentiments, concerns, and benefits reported by users [75]. For example, if a product claims to reduce wrinkles, AI can analyze customer reviews to determine if users are noticing positive changes and assess product performance across diverse consumer groups. This real-time feedback loop supplements clinical trial data and provides manufacturers with insights into how products perform in varied demographics [67, 76].

Predicting Product Effectiveness Based on Ingredient Interaction: Machine learning can help identify which ingredient combinations are most likely to produce effective results [73]. By training models on large datasets of active ingredients, formulations, and clinical outcomes, AI can predict which combinations will deliver the best anti-aging, moisturizing, or acne-fighting effects. This reduces the number of formulations that need to be tested in clinical trials, speeding up the product development process.

3.3.3 AI in mildness evaluation: Ensuring skin compatibility and sensitivity

Cosmetic mildness is crucial for ensuring consumer safety and satisfaction, particularly for individuals with sensitive skin or conditions like eczema [77]. AI can support mildness evaluation by predicting skin irritation, optimizing formulations for sensitive skin, and developing non-irritating ingredients [67, 78].

3.3.3.1 Skin irritation and sensitization prediction

Dermal Irritation Models: AI-driven models can predict whether a product will cause skin irritation by analyzing chemical properties of ingredients such as pH, molecular size, and polarity. These models use data from patch tests, human clinical trials, and historical irritation data to forecast a product's likelihood of causing irritation. By integrating these models into the product development process, AI can help manufacturers design gentler products for sensitive skin [67, 78, 79].

Skin Sensitization Prediction: AI can predict whether a product will cause allergic reactions or sensitization. Sensitization models trained on large datasets of chemical exposure and allergic responses identify substances that may trigger allergic contact dermatitis (ACD). By avoiding allergens and formulating with skin-sensitive ingredients, AI helps manufacturers create safer products for individuals with delicate skin [79].

3.3.3.2 Personalized mildness assessments

Customized Skin Care Recommendations: AI-powered platforms can assist consumers in identifying products that are best suited to their individual skin types and sensitivities. By analyzing inputs such as skin type, existing conditions (e.g., acne, rosacea), and ingredient preferences, AI algorithms can recommend products that align with individual needs. These personalized recommendations ensure that consumers use products that are both effective and gentle [80].

Real-Time Skin Sensitivity Monitoring: Emerging AI-driven wearable technologies can track changes in skin sensitivity in real-time. Wearable devices with sensors monitor parameters like skin temperature, hydration levels, and pH. The data are sent to AI-powered platforms that assess how well a product is performing, providing real-time feedback on skin sensitivity and product effectiveness [81].

3.3.4 Challenges and future directions in AI for cosmetic evaluation

While AI holds great promise for transforming cosmetic evaluation, several challenges remain. Data quality and standardization are critical, as machine learning models are only as good as the data they are trained on. Additionally, ethical concerns regarding data privacy, especially in consumer-driven applications, must be addressed. Moreover, the regulatory landscape for AI in cosmetic evaluation is still evolving, with guidelines for AI-driven tools in this industry under development [67, 68, 82, 83]. Looking ahead, advances in deep learning, natural language processing, and computer vision could revolutionize cosmetic evaluation even further. AI technologies may one day enable fully autonomous testing, from formulation design to real-time performance monitoring. This would drive innovation in the cosmetic industry while enhancing consumer safety and satisfaction [73].

3.3.4.1 Summary

The integration of AI in cosmetic evaluation is transforming how products are assessed for safety, efficacy, and mildness. By leveraging predictive models, enhancing clinical trial designs, and improving consumer insights, AI promises a more efficient, effective, and consumer-centered approach to cosmetic development. However, addressing challenges such as data quality and privacy, as well as navigating the evolving regulatory framework, will be key to fully realizing AI's potential in the cosmetic industry. As AI technologies continue to evolve, they will not only enhance product safety and effectiveness but also ensure that products are designed with consumers' individual needs and sensitivities in mind.

4. Conclusion

In the current booming cosmetics industry, the establishment of an evidence-based system for evaluating the safety and efficacy of cosmetics is of crucial importance. The cosmetic safety evaluation system constructed in the article encompasses multiple aspects such as raw materials, formulations, production processes, and products. Starting from the fundamentals like physical and chemical properties and toxicological characteristics, it employs methods such as laboratory testing, clinical trials, and risk assessment to ensure safety. Its risk assessment includes steps such as hazard identification, dose-response relationship assessment, exposure assessment, and risk characterization, ensuring accurate control of potential risks. The cosmetic efficacy evaluation system is developed for different functions. In terms of skin anti-aging, it deeply analyzes the internal and external mechanisms of skin aging and various visible signs and uses methods such as *in vitro* cell experiments and human efficacy evaluation to measure the anti-aging effects of products. For cosmetics for sensitive skin, it fully considers the differences in individual skin sensitivity, consumers' subjective experiences, and the influences of environmental and lifestyle factors.

It comprehensively conducts evaluations through subjective assessments (such as questionnaires and interviews) and objective measurements (such as patch testing and transepidermal water loss [TEWL] measurement) and ensures the safety and effectiveness of products with the help of clinical trials. Looking ahead, with the continuous innovation of technology, cutting-edge technologies such as organoids, organ-on-a-chip, and artificial intelligence will be deeply integrated. These technologies are expected to further enhance the accuracy and scientific nature of the evaluation; overcome challenges such as the safety of new raw materials, the application of nanotechnology, and the safety of personalized cosmetics; and optimize the evaluation process. It will meet consumers' increasingly diverse and personalized needs and vigorously promote the cosmetics industry to move toward a higher-quality, safer, and more reliable development stage. While safeguarding consumers' rights and interests, it will also promote the prosperity and innovation of the industry.

Author details

Li Ye[1,2]*, Jianhua Zhang[3,4], Tian Chen[5], Dongcui Li[6] and Peng Shu[7]

1 Dermatology Hospital, Southern Medical University, Guangzhou, Guangdong, China

2 Southern Medical University (NMPA Key Laboratory for Safety Evaluation of Cosmetics), Guangzhou, Guangdong, China

3 N.O.D Topia (GuangZhou) Biotechnology Co., Ltd., Guangzhou, Guangdong, China

4 Simpcare (GuangZhou) Biotechnology Co., Ltd., Guangzhou, Guangdong, China

5 Department of Environmental Health, Shanghai Municipal Center for Disease Control and Prevention, Shanghai, China

6 Hua An Tang Biotech Group Co., Ltd., Guangzhou, Guangdong, China

7 HBN Research Institute and Biological Laboratory, Shenzhen Hujia Technology Co., Ltd., Shenzhen, China

*Address all correspondence to: dlpfbyy@163.com

References

[1] SCCS. Notes of guidance for the testing of cosmetic ingredients and their safety evaluation—12th revision—European Commission. 2023. Updated. Available from: https://health.ec.europa.eu/publications/sccs-notes-guidance-testing-cosmetic-ingredients-and-their-safety-evaluation-12th-revision_en

[2] NMPA announcement on issuing the technical guidance for the safety evaluation of cosmetics. 2021. (Edition). Updated 2021. Available from: https://english.nmpa.gov.cn/2021-04/09/c_654823.html

[3] Almeida A, Sarmento B, Rodrigues F. Insights on in vitro models for safety and toxicity assessment of cosmetic ingredients. International Journal of Pharmaceutics. 2017;**519**(1-2):178-185

[4] Ficheux AS, Wesolek N, Chevillotte G, Roudot AC. Consumption of cosmetic products by the French population. First part: Frequency data. Food and Chemical Toxicology. 2015;**78**:159-169

[5] Ficheux AS, Chevillotte G, Wesolek N, et al. Consumption of cosmetic products by the French population second part: Amount data. Food and Chemical Toxicology. 2016;**90**:130-141

[6] Dornic N, Ficheux AS, Roudot AC. Consumption of cosmetic products by the French population. Third part: Product exposure amount. Food and Chemical Toxicology. 2017;**106**(Pt A):209-222

[7] Ficheux AS, Dornic N, Bernard A, Chevillotte G, Roudot AC. Probabilistic assessment of exposure to cosmetic products by French children aged 0-3 years. Food and Chemical Toxicology. 2016;**94**:85-92

[8] Gomez-Berrada M, Ficheux A, Guillou S, et al. Consumption and exposure assessment to cosmetic products for children under 2 years old. Food and Chemical Toxicology. 2017;**105**:151-160

[9] Lee E, Yun J, Ha J, et al. Assessment of exposure for baby cosmetic care products in a Korean population. Food and Chemical Toxicology. 2017;**106**(Pt A):107-113

[10] Gomez-Berrada M, Gautier F, Parent-Massin D, Ferret P. Retrospective exposure data for baby and children care products: An analysis of 48 clinical studies. Food and Chemical Toxicology. 2013;**57**:185-194

[11] Zhou L, Chen J, Chen T, et al. Investigation of actual exposure to facial sheet mask preceding its risk assessment. Scientific Reports. 2022;**12**(1):1215

[12] Hohn A et al. Happily (n)ever after: Aging in the context of oxidative stress, proteostasis loss and cellular senescence. Redox Biology. 2017;**11**:482-501

[13] Csekes E, Rackova L. Skin aging, cellular senescence and natural polyphenols. International Journal of Molecular Sciences. 2021;**22**(23):12641

[14] Jin S et al. Hallmarks of skin aging: Update. Aging and Disease. 2023;**14**(6):2167-2176

[15] Wyles SP et al. Cellular senescence in human skin aging: Leveraging senotherapeutics. Gerontology. 2024;**70**(1):7-14

[16] Lovell CR et al. Type I and III collagen content and fibre distribution in normal human skin during ageing.

The British Journal of Dermatology. 1987;**117**(4):419-428

[17] Asserin J et al. The effect of oral collagen peptide supplementation on skin moisture and the dermal collagen network: Evidence from an ex vivo model and randomized, placebo-controlled clinical trials. Journal of Cosmetic Dermatology. 2015;**14**(4):291-301

[18] Krutmann J et al. Environmentally-induced (extrinsic) skin aging: Exposomal factors and underlying mechanisms. Journal of Investigative Dermatology. 2021;**141**(4):1096-1103

[19] Gromkowska-Kępka KJ et al. The impact of ultraviolet radiation on skin photoaging—Review of in vitro studies. Journal of Cosmetic Dermatology. 2021;**20**(11):3427-3431

[20] Dong KK et al. UV-induced DNA damage initiates release of MMP-1 in human skin. Experimental Dermatology. 2008;**17**(12):1037-1044

[21] Poon F, Kang S, Chien AL. Mechanisms and treatments of photoaging. Photodermatology, Photoimmunology & Photomedicine. 2015;**31**(2):65-74

[22] Suryadevara V et al. SenNet recommendations for detecting senescent cells in different tissues. Nature Reviews. Molecular Cell Biology. 2024;**25**(12):1001-1023

[23] Lopez-Otin C et al. Hallmarks of aging: An expanding universe. Cell. 2023;**186**(2):243-278

[24] Rock K, Fischer JW. Role of the extracellular matrix in extrinsic skin aging. Der Hautarzt. 2011;**62**(8):591-597

[25] Papaccio F et al. Focus on the contribution of oxidative stress in skin aging. Antioxidants (Basel). 2022;**11**(6):1121

[26] Fernández-Varela-Gómez FA, Sandoval-García, Cabrera-Rios KV. Signs of skin aging: A review. International Journal of Research in Medical Sciences. 2024;**12**(7):2674

[27] Makrantonaki E, Bekou V, Zouboulis CC. Genetics and skin aging. Dermato-Endocrinology. 2012;**4**(3):280-284

[28] Gold M et al. Promoting a healthy skin barrier using skin care in people with mature skin xerosis. Journal of Drugs in Dermatology. 2024;**23**(1):1253-1259

[29] Foster AR et al. Osmolyte transporter expression is reduced in photoaged human skin: Implications for skin hydration in aging. Aging Cell. 2020;**19**(1):e13058

[30] Langton AK et al. A new wrinkle on old skin: The role of elastic fibres in skin ageing. International Journal of Cosmetic Science. 2010;**32**(5):330-339

[31] Bernstein EF et al. Enhanced elastin and fibrillin gene expression in chronically photodamaged skin. The Journal of Investigative Dermatology. 1994;**103**(2):182-186

[32] Passeron T et al. Clinical and biological impact of the exposome on the skin. Journal of the European Academy of Dermatology and Venereology. 2020;**34**(Suppl 4):4-25

[33] Duval C et al. A chronic pro-inflammatory environment contributes to the physiopathology of actinic lentigines. Scientific Reports. 2024;**14**(1):5256

[34] Choi W et al. Molecular and histological characterization of age

spots. Experimental Dermatology. 2017;**26**(3):242-248

[35] Kang HY et al. Alterations of the pigmentation system in the aging process. Pigment Cell & Melanoma Research. 2021;**34**(4):800-813

[36] Yoon JE et al. Senescent fibroblasts drive ageing pigmentation: A potential therapeutic target for senile lentigo. Theranostics. 2018;**8**(17):4620-4632

[37] Cruz AM et al. In vitro models for anti-aging efficacy assessment: A critical update in dermocosmetic research. Cosmetics. 2023;**10**(2):66

[38] Orimoto A et al. Transcriptome-wide profiling for melanocytes derived from newborn and adult human epidermis with enhanced proliferation. Cell Biology International. 2024;**48**(10):1573-1587

[39] Bataillon M et al. Characterization of a new reconstructed full thickness skin model, T-skin, and its application for investigations of anti-aging compounds. International Journal of Molecular Sciences. 2019;**20**(9):2240

[40] Ramasamy S et al. Optimized construction of a full thickness human skin equivalent using 3D bioprinting and a PCL/collagen dermal scaffold. Bioprinting. 2021;**21**:e00123

[41] Lombardi F et al. 3D models currently proposed to investigate human skin aging and explore preventive and reparative approaches: A descriptive review. Biomolecules. 2024;**14**(9):1066

[42] Shu P et al. Ferulic acid in synergy with retinol alleviates oxidative injury of HaCaT cells during UVB-induced photoaging. Aging (Albany NY). 2024;**16**(8):7153-7173

[43] Li WH et al. Topical stabilized retinol treatment induces the expression of HAS genes and HA production in human skin in vitro and in vivo. Archives of Dermatological Research. 2017;**309**(4):275-283

[44] Lee CM, Maibach HI. Bioengineering analysis of water hydration: An overview. Exogenous Dermatology. 2002;**1**(6):269-275

[45] Fischer TW, Wigger-Alberti W, Elsner P. Assessment of 'dry skin': Current bioengineering methods and test designs. Skin Pharmacology and Physiology. 2001;**14**(4):183-195

[46] Ivanova Z et al. Use of a novel indentometer to evaluate skin stiffness in healthy and diseased human skin. Skin Research and Technology. 2023;**29**(7):e13384

[47] Monteiro Rodrigues LJW, Fluhr, and E.G. EEMCO guidance for the in vivo assessment of biomechanical properties of the human skin and its annexes: Revisiting instrumentation and test modes. Skin Pharmacology and Physiology. 2020;**33**(1):44-60

[48] Yin Y. A New Method for Identifying Mechanical Impedence of Soft Viscoelastic Materials. 2008. Available from: https://hdl.handle.net/10356/41499

[49] Lintner K, Gerstein F, Solish N. A serum containing vitamins C & E and a matrix-repair tripeptide reduces facial signs of aging as evidenced by Primos® analysis and frequently repeated auto-perception. Journal of Cosmetic Dermatology. 2020;**19**(12):3262-3269

[50] Giovanni C, Marina PB, Tiziano Z. A retrospective 10 years- experience overview of dye laser treatments for vascular pathologies. Skin Research and Technology. 2023;**29**(8):e13427

[51] Huang YW et al. A comparative study of an advanced skin imaging system in diagnosing facial pigmentary and inflammatory conditions. Scientific Reports. 2024;**14**(1):14673

[52] Dabrowska M, Mielcarek A, Nowak I. Evaluation of sex-related changes in skin topography and structure using innovative skin testing equipment. Skin Research and Technology. 2018;**24**(4):614-620

[53] Wang H et al. Age-related morphological changes of the dermal matrix in human skin documented in vivo by multiphoton microscopy. Journal of Biomedical Optics. 2018;**23**(3):1-4

[54] Ogien J et al. Line-field confocal optical coherence tomography (LC-OCT): Principles and practical use. Italian Journal of Dermatology and Venereology. 2023;**158**(3):171-179

[55] Farage MA. The prevalence of sensitive skin. Frontiers in Medicine (Lausanne). 2019;**6**:98. DOI: 10.3389/fmed.2019.00098

[56] Misery L, Loser K, Ständer S. Sensitive skin. Journal of the European Academy of Dermatology and Venereology. 2016;**30**(Suppl 1):2-8. DOI: 10.1111/jdv.13532

[57] Misery L, Weisshaar E, Brenaut E, et al. Pathophysiology and management of sensitive skin: Position paper from the special interest group on sensitive skin of the international forum for the study of itch (IFSI). Journal of the European Academy of Dermatology and Venereology. 2020;**34**(2):222-229. DOI: 10.1111/jdv.16000

[58] Misery L, Jean-Decoster C, Mery S, Georgescu V, Sibaud V. A new ten-item questionnaire for assessing sensitive skin: The sensitive Scale-10. Acta Dermato-Venereologica. 2014;**94**(6):635-639. DOI: 10.2340/00015555-1870

[59] Corazza M, Guarneri F, Montesi L, Toni G, Donelli I, Borghi A. Proposal of a self-assessment questionnaire for the diagnosis of sensitive skin. Journal of Cosmetic Dermatology. 2022;**21**(6):2488-2496. DOI: 10.1111/jocd.14425

[60] Finlay AY, Khan GK. Dermatology life quality index (DLQI)--A simple practical measure for routine clinical use. Clinical and Experimental Dermatology. 1994;**19**(3):210-216. DOI: 10.1111/j.1365-2230.1994.tb01167.x

[61] Chee SN, Murrell D. A comparison of dermatology life quality index scores in a dermatology practice setting. Journal of the American Academy of Dermatology. 2009;**Supplement 1**:AB94. DOI: 10.1016/j.jaad.2008.11.420

[62] Kumar P, Paulose R. Patch testing in suspected allergic contact dermatitis to cosmetics. Dermatology Research and Practice. 2014;**2014**:695387. DOI: 10.1155/2014/695387

[63] Cho HJ, Chung BY, Lee HB, Kim HO, Park CW, Lee CH. Quantitative study of stratum corneum ceramides contents in patients with sensitive skin. The Journal of Dermatology. 2012;**39**(3):295-300. DOI: 10.1111/j.1346-8138.2011.01406.x

[64] Green M, Kashetsky N, Feschuk A, Maibach HI. Transepidermal water loss (TEWL): Environment and pollution-a systematic review. Skin Health and Disease. 2022;**2**(2):e104. Published 2022 Feb 25. DOI: 10.1002/ski2.104

[65] Pan Y, Ma X, Song Y, Zhao J, Yan S. Questionnaire and lactic acid sting test play different role on the assessment of sensitive skin: A cross-sectional study. Clinical, Cosmetic and Investigational

Dermatology. 2021;**14**:1215-1225. DOI: 10.2147/CCID.S325166

[66] Zhang J, Liu S, Guo W, Li N, Huang Y. A highly efficient and user-friendly sensitive skin model on the forearm. Journal of Cosmetic Dermatology. 2024;**0**:1-10. DOI: 10.1111/jocd.16619

[67] Vatiwutipong P, Vachmanus S, Noraset T. Artificial intelligence in cosmetic dermatology: A systematic literature review. IEEE Access. 2023;**11**:71407-71425. DOI: 10.1109/ACCESS.2023.3295001

[68] Jayanthy G, Majumdar A, Kaloo S. Enhancing patient safety: Leveraging artificial intelligence-powered electronic medical records for effective drug-drug interaction nudge in real-world prescribing practices. International Journal of Basic & Clinical Pharmacology. 2024;**13**(4):520-525. DOI: 10.18203/2319-2003.ijbcp20241653

[69] Nilsen P, David S, Heintz F. Towards evidence-based practice 2.0: Leveraging artificial intelligence in healthcare. Frontiers in Health Services. 2024;**4**:1368030. DOI: 10.3389/frhs.2024.1368030

[70] Rudroff T. Artificial intelligence as a replacement for animal experiments in neurology: Potential, Progress, and challenges. Neurology International. 2024;**16**:805-820. DOI: 10.3390/neurolint16040060

[71] Cavasotto CN, Scardino V. Machine learning toxicity prediction: Latest advances by toxicity end point. ACS Omega. 2022;7:47536-47546. DOI: 10.1021/acsomega.2c05693

[72] Tonoyan L, Siraki AG. Machine learning in toxicological sciences: Opportunities for assessing drug toxicity. Frontiers in Drug Discovery. 2024:4. DOI: 10.3389/fddsv.2024.1336025

[73] Elder A, Ring C, Heitmiller K. The role of artificial intelligence in cosmetic dermatology-current, upcoming, and future trends. Journal of Cosmetic Dermatology. 2021;**20**(1):48-52. DOI: 10.1111/jocd.13797

[74] Haykal D. Harnessing AI in laser aesthetic treatments: Revolutionizing precision, safety, and personalization. Journal of Cosmetic Dermatology. 2024;**0**:e16704. DOI: 10.1111/jocd.16704

[75] Frank K, Day D, Few J. AI assistance in aesthetic medicine-a consensus on objective medical standards. Journal of Cosmetic Dermatology. 2024;**23**(12):4110-4115. DOI: 10.1111/jocd.16481

[76] Cummins JA, Nambudiri VE. Natural language processing: A window to understanding skincare trends. International Journal of Medical Informatics. 2022;**160**:104705. DOI: 10.1016/j.ijmedinf.2022.104705. Epub 2022 Jan 24

[77] Ennen J, Degwert J, Duttiné M. Studies on the skin compatibility of cosmetics involving human subjects-study portfolio and test strategy. IFSCC Magazine. 2016;**1**(17):19-23

[78] Rehman AU, Li MY, Wu BJ. Role of artificial intelligence in revolutionizing drug discovery. Fundamental Research. 2024;**11**(30):807-810. DOI: 10.1016/j.fmre.2024.04.021

[79] Kalicińska J, Wiśniowska B, Polak S. Artificial intelligence that predicts sensitizing potential of cosmetic ingredients with accuracy comparable to animal and In vitro tests—How does the infotechnomics compare to other "omics" in the cosmetics safety assessment?

International Journal of Molecular Sciences. 2023;**24**(7):6801. DOI: 10.3390/ijms24076801

[80] Stern C. How AI-Powered Beauty Delivers Hyper-Personalized Products & Sustainable Solutions in Real Time [Internet]. 2024. Available from: https://www.cosmeticsdesign.com/Article/2024/09/11/long-read-how-ai-powered-beauty-delivers-hyper-personalized-products-sustainable-solutions-in-real-time/

[81] Shajari S, Kuruvinashetti K, Komeili A. The emergence of AI-based wearable sensors for digital health technology: A review. Sensors. 2023;**23**:9498. DOI: 10.3390/ s23239498

[82] Li YH, Li YL, Wei MY. Innovation and challenges of artificial intelligence technology in personalized healthcare. Scientific Reports. 2024;**14**:18994. DOI: 10.1038/s41598-024-70073-7

[83] Drabiak K. Leveraging law and ethics to promote safe and reliable AI/ML in healthcare. Frontiers in Nuclear Medicine. 2022;**27**(2):983340. DOI: 10.3389/fnume.2022.983340

Chapter 4

Applications of Plant-Based Materials in Cosmetics

Yuchao Tang and Xiaoqin Wang

Abstract

Cosmetics have become indispensable in modern life, which lead to increasing attention being paid to their ingredient sources and safety. Plant-based materials are generally regarded as safer and gentle, making them suitable for sensitive skin. These materials typically lack synthetic chemicals, thereby reducing the risk of allergic reactions and irritation. At the same time, plant ingredients are often rich in essential nutrients and natural antioxidants, providing nourishment to the skin and promoting overall skin health. Moreover, plant-based materials are produced sustainably, which minimizes their environmental impact and aligns with eco-friendly principles. Additionally, plant-derived substances, such as essential oils, not only enhance the fragrance of cosmetics but also contribute to relaxation and improved user experience. In summary, plant-based materials are indispensable contributors to the health and sustainable development of cosmetic products.

Keywords: cosmetics, plant-based material, bioactive compound, essential oil, antioxidant, skin care, antimicrobial

1. Introduction

With the improvement in living standards, people's pursuit of beauty has become increasingly focused on quality and details, with growing attention to personal appearance. This has driven the cosmetics industry to become one of the most important and fastest-growing sectors in the global economy [1]. The skin, as the largest organ of the human body, is also the most prominent area of focus in the cosmetics industry. It serves not only as the external protective barrier of the body but also as a vital component of one's appearance. Healthy skin can boost self-confidence and contribute to mental well-being. Frequently, the skin (such as the face and hands) is directly exposed to the external environment, making it vulnerable to damage or suboptimal health. Moreover, in recent years, the skin has been recognized as an important route for drug delivery [2]. Therefore, if harmful substances are present in cosmetics, they can easily penetrate the body, posing potential health risks. For example, per- and polyfluoroalkyl substances (PFAS) are used in cosmetics due to their excellent hydrophobicity and film-forming properties, enhancing durability and waterproofing. It is claimed that PFAS can increase skin absorption of the products, improving skin appearance or texture. However, many cosmetics (such as sunscreens and lipsticks) are applied directly to areas near the eyes and mouth, potentially increasing exposure and absorption, which in turn raises the risk of ingestion [3]. As a result, an increasing number of consumers are becoming concerned about the safety of cosmetic ingredients, with a growing demand for products containing natural ingredients.

Plant-based materials refer to various substances or ingredients extracted or obtained from plants. These materials can be sourced from different parts of plants, such as roots, stems, leaves, flowers, and fruits. Plant-based materials include plant oils, essential oils, phenolic acids, flavonoids, alkaloids, peptides, polysaccharides, and others [4]. At the same time, plant-based materials are typically gentle and possess natural properties, which help reduce the irritation and allergic reactions caused by synthetic chemicals on the skin. For example, plant oils and plant extracts are widely used in skincare products due to their excellent moisturizing, anti-inflammatory, and antioxidant effects [5]. With the growing concern over the safety and health of cosmetics, the use of plant-based materials better meets consumers' demand for harmless, natural, and healthy products. Additionally, in the context of the ongoing global environmental crisis and resource scarcity, plant-based materials not only provide sustainable solutions for the cosmetics industry but also cater to consumers' increasing demand for natural, healthy, and eco-friendly products. As technology advances and the demand for green products continues to rise, the application of plant-based materials is expected to play an increasingly significant role in the cosmetics industry.

This chapter provides an overview of the advantages of plant-based materials, as well as their applications and benefits in cosmetics. It further analyzes the current status and challenges of plant-based materials in cosmetics and offers insights into the future prospects and directions for their application in this field.

2. The advantages of plant-based materials

2.1 Wide range of resources

Plants are a core component of the Earth's ecosystem and one of the essential resources of materials that sustain human life. The range of plant sources that can be used as cosmetic ingredients is vast, encompassing various plant tissues, including roots, stems, leaves, flowers, fruits, and seeds. Common flowers such as rose [6], lily [7], and lavender [8], vegetables like cucumber [9], carrot [10], asparagus [11], and broccoli [12], fruits such as lemon [13, 14], apple [15], and grape [16], as well as other plants like tea [17] and aloe vera [18], can all serve as natural sources for cosmetic ingredients.

2.2 Rich in ingredients and diverse in functions

Plants are rich in various bioactive molecules, such as amino acids, vitamins, phenolics, flavonoids, polysaccharides, and peptides, which serve as natural nutrients for the skin. These components can effectively nourish the skin, scavenge free radicals, whiten, repair skin damage, and delay aging, among other benefits [4]. Furthermore, plant-based ingredients, derived from natural plants, typically do not contain irritating substances and are relatively mild, making them suitable for all skin types, especially sensitive skin [5]. Some plant-derived ingredients also possess soothing and anti-inflammatory properties, thus enhancing safety and effectively reducing the risk of allergic reactions.

2.3 Gentle in nature and good biocompatibility

Plant-derived ingredients typically exhibit good compatibility with the biological structure and functions of the human body, allowing them to interact gently with the skin and promote skin health without causing adverse reactions or allergies. Components, such as plant fatty acids, plant oils, and plant proteins, can help repair the skin and restore its natural barrier function, alleviating discomfort. For example, plant oils can penetrate deep into the skin, providing long-lasting moisture without leaving a greasy feeling, thereby maintaining the skin's oil-water balance.

2.4 Sustainable and eco-friendly

As global environmental issues continue to intensify, the sustainable development of the cosmetic industry has become a critical topic. Plant-based materials, derived from renewable resources, not only reduce reliance on non-renewable resources [1], but most of them are also biodegradable, preventing long-term environmental pollution. As a result, plant-based materials are gradually becoming an eco-friendly and green alternative in the cosmetics industry, aligning with the principles of sustainable and green development.

From the perspective of cosmetic ingredient sources, plant-based materials are diverse, widely available, nutritionally comprehensive, mild in composition, and biologically compatible, with the added benefits of sustainability and environmental friendliness. These attributes make plant-based materials an increasingly popular choice in the cosmetic industry, especially as consumers place greater emphasis on environmental protection, health, and natural ingredients. With advancements in technology, the extraction processes and efficacy of plant-based ingredients have continuously improved, offering the cosmetics industry more innovation and potential.

3. Functions of plant-based materials in cosmetics

3.1 Antioxidant

Free radicals can lead to skin aging and damage, making antioxidant properties particularly important in cosmetic products. Both external factors (such as ultraviolet (UV) radiation, air pollution, etc.) and internal factors (such as metabolism and aging) can trigger the formation of unstable molecules. These free radicals can damage skin cells, resulting in issues, such as skin aging, pigmentation, and fine lines [19]. Plant-based materials contain rich natural antioxidants, such as vitamins, phenolic acids, flavonoids, and polysaccharides, which can effectively neutralize free radicals, reduce oxidative damage to the skin, and have anti-aging and skin-aging-delaying effects.

Numerous studies have already confirmed the powerful free radical scavenging ability and anti-aging effects of plant-based materials, making them a widespread source of antioxidants in cosmetics [20]. Test results based on ferric reducing antioxidant power (FRAP), 2,2-diphenyl-1-picrylhydrazyl (DPPH), oxygen radical absorption capacity (ORAC), and photochemiluminescence (PCL) assays show that

Moringa oleifera leaf extracts, rich in phenolic compounds, represent a promising source of cosmetic ingredients with potential anti-aging and oxidative stress-reducing properties for skin [21]. Moreover, experiments have demonstrated that extracts from lily bulbs, rich in phenolic acids and flavonoids, exhibit excellent in vitro antioxidant properties, making them a potential cosmetic ingredient [22]. Face masks developed from olive pomace, rich in vitamin E and phenolic substances, show strong antioxidant activity [23].

3.2 Anti-inflammatory

Skin damage can be caused by either intrinsic diseases or the immune system's excessive response to external stimuli, such as infections, injuries, or allergic reactions. If not effectively controlled or treated, these responses may lead to a range of skin issues, affecting both the appearance and function of the skin. Many plant-derived compounds, such as polyphenols, flavonoids, triterpenes, and polysaccharides, possess natural anti-inflammatory properties. Plant extracts from *Betulae*, *Liquiritiae*, and *Avenae* exhibit excellent antioxidant characteristics, and at low doses, these extracts can exert anti-inflammatory effects by enhancing cell migration under oxidative stress-related inflammatory conditions [24]. A retrospective review suggests that the circumpolar plant *Epilobium angustifolium* offers potential for cosmetic formulations with skin-conditioning and anti-inflammatory properties [25]. Additionally, many essential oils from plants are effective natural anti-inflammatory agents. For example, the active ingredients in *Mentha piperita*, *Rosmarinus officinalis*, and *Lavandula officinalis* essential oils are commonly used as antioxidants and anti-inflammatory agents to provide skin protection [26].

3.3 Antimicrobial

Antimicrobial properties are essential for the safety, efficacy, and user experience of cosmetic products, as they help protect the skin from infections and extend the shelf life of the products. Plant-derived compounds, such as polyphenols, alkaloids, saponins, and essential oils, are important antimicrobial ingredients. Existing studies have demonstrated that plants, such as *Olea europaea*, *Melaleuca alternifolia* var. *alternifolia*, *Eucalyptus globulus*, *Thymus vulgaris*, and *Cinnamomum zeylanicum*, are significant natural sources of antimicrobial substances [27, 28]. The inclusion of these natural extracts not only enhances the antimicrobial properties of cosmetics but also provides additional benefits, such as antioxidant and anti-inflammatory functions, making them more favored by consumers. Moreover, the use of these substances helps avoid the application of synthetic antimicrobial agents, ensuring both product safety and achieving environmental sustainability goals.

3.4 Photoprotection

Photoprotection is a critical indicator of the quality of cosmetics, particularly sunscreen products. It effectively protects the skin from ultraviolet (UV) damage, delays aging, reduces skin lesions, and helps maintain healthy, even skin tone. Certain natural ingredients in plant-based materials can enhance the skin's natural barrier function, improving its ability to resist external stimuli and environmental damage. Plant-derived compounds, rich in flavonoids, carotenoids, and polysaccharides, are effective at absorbing UV radiation, thereby reducing the impact of light exposure on the skin [29]. Additionally, many plant-derived active ingredients can effectively scavenge free radicals induced by radiation, further contributing to skin protection [30].

3.5 Skin whitening

In addition to their strong photoprotective properties, plant-derived chemical compounds can also inhibit melanin production and improve uneven skin tone, thereby achieving a whitening effect. For instance, *Portulaca oleracea* polysaccharide VPOP3 exhibits excellent anti-photoaging and anti-melanin synthesis activities [31]. Herbal extracts, as potential multi-target agents for photoprotection, tyrosinase inhibition, and skin whitening, have shown promise in treating hyperpigmentation [32]. Herbs, such as licorice, rhubarb, sorrel, and olive, have positive effects on melasma treatment [33]. Polysaccharides from *Bletilla striata* provide protection against ultraviolet B (UVB)-induced skin oxidative stress and exhibit tyrosinase inhibition [34, 35]. *Litsea cubeba* essential oil demonstrates strong inhibition of tyrosinase and melanin production, suggesting its potential as a promising natural ingredient for skin whitening in cosmetics [36].

3.6 Skin repairing

Allergic reactions, trauma, infections, and the aging process can lead to skin damage. By repairing the skin's healthy barrier and promoting skin regeneration, these processes not only improve skin texture and appearance but also delay the aging process and enhance overall skin health. Research has shown that many plant-derived compounds possess skin repair and wound healing properties. On one hand, plant-based ingredients can prevent infected skin by exerting antioxidant, anti-inflammatory, and antimicrobial effects. On the other hand, these compounds can promote cell proliferation by regulating the metabolic pathways of skin cells, thus facilitating skin repair and reducing scarring [37]. For example, *Aralia elata* flower essential oil has been shown to promote skin cell proliferation and the production of type IV collagen, thereby achieving skin repair [38].

3.7 Moisturizing

Decreased skin moisture content and increased water dispersion lead to dry skin, which can trigger symptoms such as scaling, itching, and cracking, severely affecting both skin health and appearance. Many plant extracts exhibit moisturizing effects. On one hand, components such as polysaccharides, fatty acids, and waxes in plant preparations can form a barrier on the skin surface, effectively preventing moisture loss. On the other hand, the active ingredients in plants can nourish the skin, promoting its health and thereby effectively locking in moisture. Studies have shown that the use of plant formulations rich in polysaccharides can produce a moisturizing effect by promoting the expression of the filaggrin (FLG) and claudin 1 (CLDN-1) genes and increasing the accumulation of aquaporin 3 (AQP3) proteins [39]. Extracts of *Prosopis juliflora*, rich in α-glucans and phenolic compounds, also demonstrate excellent potential for skin hydration and microrelief improvement [40].

It is important to note that due to the complex and diverse nature of plant preparations, the effects mentioned above are not singular. The same plant-based materials often exhibit multiple functions in cosmetics, a multifunctionality that has been extensively studied. For example, *Ammodaucus leucotrichus* essential oil simultaneously possesses potent antibacterial, antioxidant, and anti-inflammatory activities [41]. Rosehip-based dermatological products exhibit multiple benefits, including promoting wound healing, enhancing collagen synthesis, treating atopic dermatitis, alleviating melasma, and offering anti-aging effects [42].

4. Current status of plant-based materials in cosmetics

To fully understand the current status of the application of plant-based materials in cosmetics, we conducted a bibliometric analysis of academic papers on this topic using the Web of Science Core Collection. After several attempts, we selected the following keywords for thematic search: (plant) AND ((essential oil) OR (extract) OR (hydrolat) OR (polypeptide) OR (polysaccharide) OR (plant oil)) AND (cosmetic) (accessed on February 06, 2025). After excluding other document types, we retained only "Article" type, resulting in a total of 3276 papers for subsequent analysis. The relevant data were analyzed and visualized using Excel Office and VOSviewer software.

4.1 The research development of plant-based materials in cosmetics has been advancing rapidly

Interestingly, although the use of natural ingredients in cosmetics can be traced back to approximately 3000 B.C. [43], academic publications on the components and effects of plant-based materials in cosmetics have only emerged in recent decades. The number of publications gradually increased from fewer than 10 per year in the early 2000s to over 100 per year by 2013 (**Figure 1A**). Notably, these data saw a rapid increase from 2019 to 2022, nearly doubling during this period, and then stabilized at over 400 papers per year. This indicates that research on the application of plant-based materials in cosmetics is currently at a historical peak. In terms of publishing countries/regions, China leads in the number of publications, followed by India, Brazil, Italy, and Poland (**Figure 1B**).

It is important to note that although there are currently only about 3000 academic papers on the components and effects of plant-based materials in cosmetics, the attempts to apply plant-based materials in cosmetics are far more extensive. Some researchers and companies have sought intellectual property protection by patenting the product formulations they have developed. It has been reported that between 56.6 and 94% of the content in patents across various industries worldwide has never been published in other forms, including in scientific papers [44]. Additionally, there are tens of thousands of plant-based cosmetic products on the market, further highlighting the significant role of plant-based materials in cosmetic production.

4.2 The functionality, composition, and safety of plant-based materials have garnered widespread attention

Co-occurrence analysis grouped keywords with a frequency of ≥20 into five clusters (**Figure 2**). In functional descriptions, "antioxidant" appeared most frequently, making it the central node, followed by "antimicrobial." Additionally, "tyrosinase inhibition" also garnered significant attention. In ingredient-related descriptions, "extracts," "essential oil," and "bioactive compounds" occupy core positions, while "phenolics," "flavonoids," and "plant oil" are also widely discussed. Furthermore,

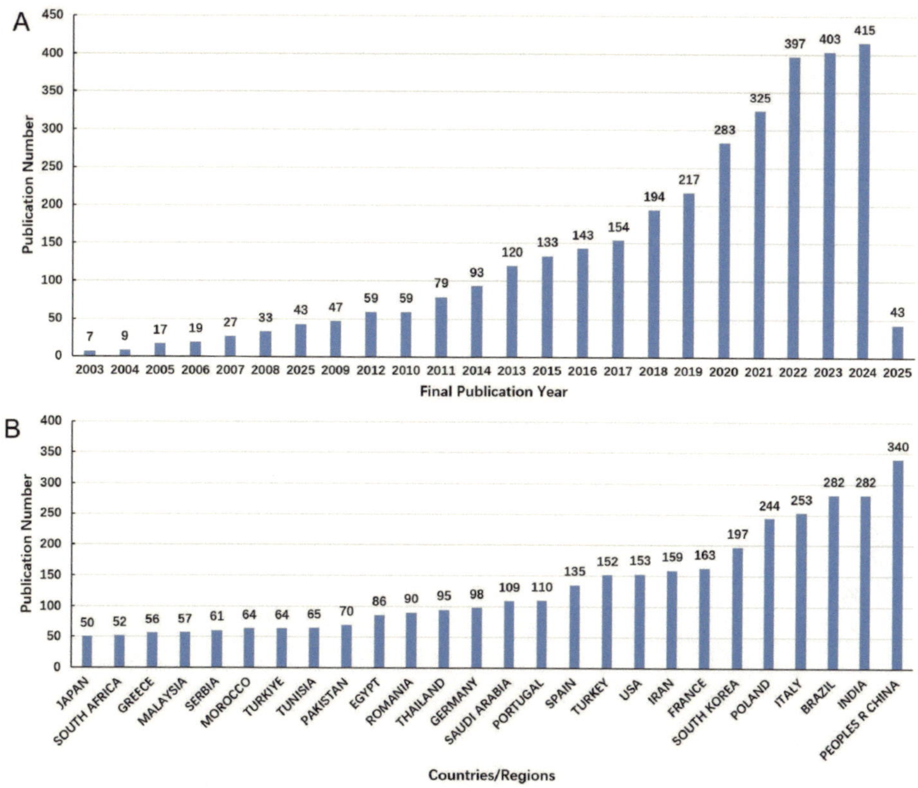

Figure 1.
The number of research papers on the application of plant-based materials in cosmetics published in different years (A) and the countries/regions with over 50 published papers (B).

several key nodes are noteworthy, such as "medicinal plant," which aligns with the current pursuit of cosmeceuticals, and the widespread attention to "toxicity," reflecting the growing emphasis on the safety of cosmetic products.

5. Challenges and future perspectives

Thanks to their natural, safe, and low side-effect characteristics, plant-based materials are becoming increasingly prevalent in cosmetic applications. However, several safety issues and challenges remain during their use. These issues include potential allergic reactions to plant ingredients, unknown toxicity, incomplete related regulations, and a lack of products suitable for special populations. Although plant-based foods are common in our daily diet, a recent review indicated that approximately 40% of raw materials used in the production of plant-based foods contain various allergenic compounds [45]. The flower extract of *Ipomoea horsfalliae* not only demonstrates excellent photoprotective effects, but also exhibits significant fibroblast cytotoxicity [46]. Additionally, natural banana starch nanoparticles may pose health risks by compromising the integrity of the intestinal barrier [47]. These findings suggest that even though plant-based materials are generally considered mild, they can still provoke potential allergic reactions. Moreover, due to the specific physiological characteristics of certain populations (such as pregnant women, infants,

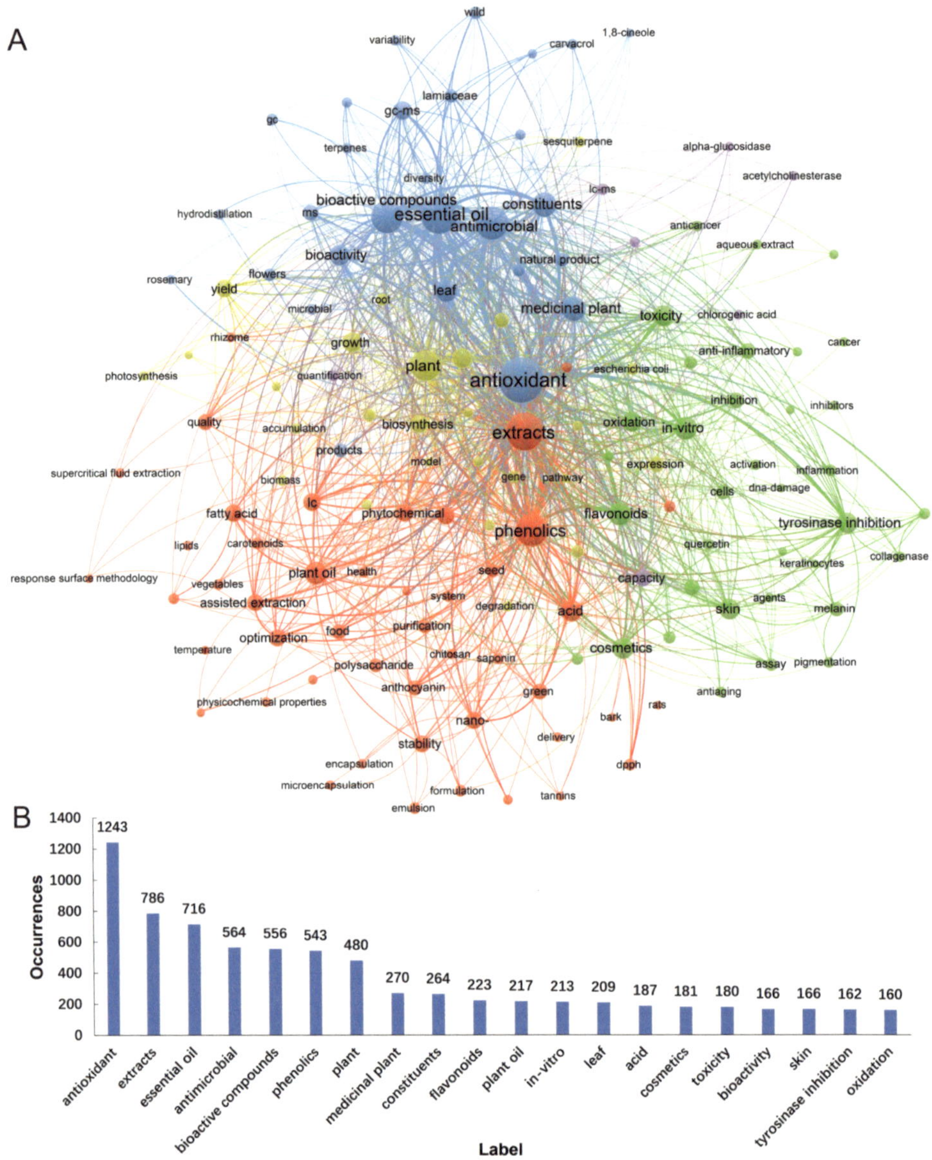

Figure 2.
Co-occurrence analysis of keyword frequencies in research papers on the application of plant-based materials in cosmetics (frequency ≥ 20) (A) and the top 20 ranked nodes by frequency (B).

and the elderly), common cosmetic ingredients may not achieve the expected effects and could even lead to adverse consequences [48]. As the ingredients in cosmetics become increasingly complex and diverse, the difficulty of evaluating and managing their safety is growing, making the formulation and refinement of relevant laws and regulations even more urgent [49].

In conclusion, the application of plant-based materials in cosmetics has become a significant trend in the current beauty industry. With the increasing consumer focus on health, environmental sustainability, and natural ingredients, plant-based materials, due to their natural, gentle, and eco-friendly properties, are gradually becoming the core components in cosmetic product formulations. Based on the current status and challenges of plant-based materials in cosmetics, future research in this field will focus more on aspects such as the sourcing of raw materials, functional exploration, personalized product development, safety assessments, and regulatory frameworks, in order to achieve the healthy and sustainable development of the cosmetic industry.

1. Expansion of plant material sources: Ethnobotanical plants are a crucial reservoir of natural ingredients. On one hand, the potential of these plants in cosmetic products should be thoroughly evaluated; on the other hand, more efforts should be made to utilize plant resources that grow in harsh environments, as their production typically does not compete with major food crop spaces. In the context of global food shortages, if these plants can be developed, they would not only avoid impacting the production of staple food and economic crops but also create new, more competitive products, which could further stimulate local economic development. Additionally, fermenting existing plant resources to enhance the content of active ingredients and using tissue or cell cultures for the preparation of plant-based materials are promising directions for future research.

2. Exploration of physiological functions of plant-based materials: Powerful functions serve as a critical theoretical foundation for the successful promotion of cosmetic products. Using modern physiological, biochemical, and molecular biology techniques to explore and validate the functions of compounds can effectively increase product acceptability among consumers and facilitate the development of new cosmetic products for specific applications or scenarios.

3. Personalized product development: In the development of personalized cosmetic products, it is essential to fully consider the needs and characteristics of different age groups, genders, skin types, and special populations. Targeted cosmetic formulations should be provided to meet the demands of a broader consumer base. Additionally, with the increasing self-awareness among individuals today, personalized product customization represents a new avenue for the development of specialized cosmetic products.

4. Development of emerging products: With the growing emphasis on health and natural care, there has been a continuous increase in demand for multifunctional and comprehensive cosmetic products. This has led to the emergence of terms such as *Cosmeceuticals* and *Nutricosmetics*. *Cosmeceuticals* refer to products that offer both cosmetic benefits and therapeutic functions, while *Nutricosmetics* reflects the concept of improving skin health through the supplementation of specific nutrients. The emergence of these new terms reflects emerging trends within the beauty industry, providing fresh insights and directions for cosmetic manufacturers to develop more competitive products.

5. Product safety assessment: While plant-based materials are relatively safe, they still carry potential risks of allergens or even toxicity. Furthermore, during the production of plant materials, there may be risks such as pesticide residues or heavy metal accumulation. Therefore, a thorough safety assessment of raw materials is an essential step. Concurrently, relevant structures should establish and improve legal regulations and management practices based on specific circumstances, ensuring the safety of cosmetic products.

Acknowledgements

We gratefully acknowledge the funding of this study by the Postdoctoral Fellowship Program of China Postdoctoral Science Foundation (GZC20230248) and The Open Research Program from the Research Center for Cooperation and Development between Xinjiang, China, and Neighboring Countries (2021ZBGJYB008).

Conflict of interest

The authors declare no conflict of interest.

Author details

Yuchao Tang[1*] and Xiaoqin Wang[2*]

1 National Engineering Research Center for Floriculture, School of Landscape Architecture, Beijing Forestry University, Beijing, China

2 Key Laboratory of Plant Resources Protection and Utilization in Xinjiang Yili Valley, College of Biological Science and Technology, Yili Normal University, Yili, China

*Address all correspondence to: tangyucha100@126.com
and xiaoqinwang@ylnu.edu.cn

References

[1] Mondello A, Salomone R, Mondello G. Exploring circular economy in the cosmetic industry: Insights from a literature review. Environmental Impact Assessment Review. 2024;**105**:107443

[2] Saeedi M, Eslamifar M, Khezri K. Kojic acid applications in cosmetic and pharmaceutical preparations. Biomedicine and Pharmacotherapy. 2019;**110**:582-593

[3] Whitehead HD, Venier M, Wu Y, et al. Fluorinated compounds in north American cosmetics. Environmental Science and Technology Letters. 2021;**8**(7):538-544

[4] Samtiya M, Aluko RE, Dhewa T, et al. Potential health benefits of plant food-derived bioactive components: An overview. Food. 2021;**10**(4):839

[5] Michalak M. Plant extracts as skin care and therapeutic agents. International Journal of Molecular Sciences. 2023;**24**(20):15444

[6] Sallustio V, Rossi M, Marto J, et al. Green extraction of *Rosa canina L.* and *Prunus spinosa L.* by NaDES and their encapsulation in chitosan nanoparticles for cosmetic industry. Industrial Crops and Products. 2024;**218**:119042

[7] Tang Y, Liu Y, Luo K, et al. Potential applications of lilium plants in cosmetics: A comprehensive review based on research papers and patents. Antioxidants. 2022;**11**(8):1458

[8] Lesage-Meessen L, Bou M, Sigoillot JC, et al. Essential oils and distilled straws of lavender and lavandin: A review of current use and potential application in white biotechnology. Applied Microbiology and Biotechnology. 2015;**99**:3375-3385

[9] Vats M, Bhardwaj S, Chhabra A. Green synthesis of copper oxide nanoparticles using Cucumis sativus (cucumber) extracts and their bio-physical and biochemical characterization for cosmetic and dermatologic applications. Endocrine, Metabolic and Immune Disorders-Drug Targets (Formerly Current Drug Targets-Immune, Endocrine and Metabolic Disorders). 2021;**21**(4):726-733

[10] Kurzawa M, Wilczyńska E, Brudzyńska P, et al. Total phenolic content, antioxidant capacity and UV radiation protection properties of marigold (*Calendula officinalis*), carrot (*Daucus carota*), tomato (*Solanum lycopersicum*) and hop (*Humulus lupulus*) extracts. Cosmetics. 2022;**9**(6):134

[11] Ginting HS, Fachrial E, Lister INE, et al. Anti-aging activities of asparagus gel ethanol extract in cosmetic gel agent for facial skin. Majalah Kedokteran Bandung. 2021;**53**(3):119-125

[12] Borja-Martínez M, Lozano-Sánchez J, Borrás-Linares I, et al. Revalorization of broccoli by-products for cosmetic uses using supercritical fluid extraction. Antioxidants. 2020;**9**(12):1195

[13] Klimek-Szczykutowicz M, Szopa A, Ekiert H. Citrus Limon (lemon) phenomenon—A review of the chemistry, pharmacological properties, applications in the modern pharmaceutical, food, and cosmetics industries, and biotechnological studies. Plants. 2020;**9**(1):119

[14] Leong EJ, Tan LF, Yap VL, et al. Cosmetological applications of Citrus Limon: A mini-review. Indian Journal of Natural Products and Resources (IJNPR) [Formerly Natural Product Radiance (NPR)]. 2024;**15**(2):286-293

[15] Vandorou M, Plakidis C, Tsompanidou IM, et al. A review on apple pomace bioactives for natural functional food and cosmetic products with therapeutic health-promoting properties. International Journal of Molecular Sciences. 2024;**25**(19): 10856

[16] Michailidis D, Angelis A, Nikolaou PE, et al. Exploitation of vitis vinifera, foeniculum vulgare, cannabis sativa and punica granatum by-product seeds as dermo-cosmetic agents. Molecules. 2021;**26**(3):731

[17] Messire G, Serreau R, Berteina-Raboin S. Antioxidant effects of catechins (EGCG), andrographolide, and curcuminoids compounds for skin protection, cosmetics, and dermatological uses: An update. Antioxidants. 2023;**12**(7):1317

[18] Lee ZM, Goh BH, Khaw KY. Aloe vera and the proliferative phase of cutaneous wound healing: Status quo report on active principles, mechanisms, and applications. Planta Medica. 2025;**91**:4-18

[19] Young AR, Claveau J, Rossi AB. Ultraviolet radiation and the skin: Photobiology and sunscreen photoprotection. Journal of the American Academy of Dermatology. 2017;**76**(3):S100-S109

[20] Choi HY, Lee YJ, Kim CM, et al. Revolutionizing cosmetic ingredients: Harnessing the power of antioxidants, probiotics, plant extracts, and peptides in personal and skin care products. Cosmetics. 2024;**11**(5):157

[21] Baldisserotto A, Barbari R, Tupini C, et al. Multifunctional profiling of Moringa oleifera leaf extracts for topical application: A comparative study of different collection time. Antioxidants. 2023;**12**(2):411

[22] Tang YC, Liu YJ, He GR, et al. Comprehensive analysis of secondary metabolites in the extracts from different lily bulbs and their antioxidant ability. Antioxidants. 2021;**10**(10):1634

[23] Rodrigues R, Lobo JC, Ferreira DM, et al. Chemical and rheological characterization of a facial mask containing an olive pomace fraction. Cosmetics. 2023;**10**(2):64

[24] Ghica A, Tănase ML, Niculițe CM, et al. In vitro toxicity evaluation of some plant extracts and their potential application in Xerosis cutis. Cosmetics. 2024;**11**(4):124

[25] Ailus J, Saleem I, Ismail FMD. A review of the anti-inflammatory skincare potential of *Epilobium angustifolium* (fireweed) inspired by herbal tradition. Cosmetics. 2024;**11**(5):156

[26] Guzmán E, Lucia A. Essential oils and their individual components in cosmetic products. Cosmetics. 2021;**8**(4):114

[27] Magyari-Pavel IZ, Moacă EA, Avram Ș, et al. Antioxidant extracts from Greek and Spanish olive leaves: Antimicrobial, anticancer and antiangiogenic effects. Antioxidants. 2024;**13**(7):774

[28] Rybczyńska-Tkaczyk K, Grenda A, Jakubczyk A, et al. Natural compounds with antimicrobial properties in cosmetics. Pathogens. 2023;**12**(2):320

[29] Cefali LC, Ataide JA, Moriel P, et al. Plant-based active photoprotectants for sunscreens. International Journal of Cosmetic Science. 2016;**38**(4):346-353

[30] Shubayr N. Phytochemicals properties of herbal extracts for ultraviolet protection and skin health:

A narrative review. Journal of Radiation Research and Applied Sciences. 2023;**16**(4):100729

[31] Tao X, Hu X, Wu T, et al. Characterization and screening of anti-melanogenesis and anti-photoaging activity of different enzyme-assisted polysaccharide extracts from *Portulaca oleracea L*. Phytomedicine. 2023;**116**:154879

[32] Kothapalli L, Bhosale K, Thomas A, et al. Potential of herbal extracts as sunscreens and antihyperpigmentation treatment. Current Drug Therapy. 2023;**18**(5):377-390

[33] Kumari M, Sadhu P, Shah N, et al. The science of skin ageing: From radicals to herbal remedies. Annals of Phytomedicine. 2024;**13**(1):108-117

[34] Chen H, Wu Y, Wang B, et al. Skin healthcare protection with antioxidant and anti-melanogenesis activity of polysaccharide purification from Bletilla striata. International Journal of Biological Macromolecules. 2024;**262**:130016

[35] Chen H, Lin C, Wu Y, et al. Protective effects of degraded Bletilla striata polysaccharides against UVB-induced oxidative stress in skin. International Journal of Biological Macromolecules. 2024;**277**:134462

[36] Qiu Y, Wang Y, Li Y. Solvent-free microwave extraction of essential oils from *Litsea cubeba* (Lour.) Pers. at different harvesting times and their skin-whitening cosmetic potential. Antioxidants. 2022;**11**(12):2389

[37] Ti YL, Song F, Fang Z, et al. Plants and phytochemicals inhibit scar formation: A systematic review. Industrial Crops and Products. 2022;**185**:115113

[38] Kim DY, Won KJ, Kim YY, et al. Potential wound healing and anti-melanogenic activities in skin cells of Aralia elata (Miq.) Seem. Flower Essential Oil and Its Chemical Composition. Pharmaceutics. 2024;**16**(8):1008

[39] Meng H, Li J, Dong Y, et al. Poly traditional Chinese medicine formulation prepared with skin moisturizing properties. Dermatologic Therapy. 2020;**33**(6):e14105

[40] Damasceno GAB, Barreto SMAG, Reginaldo FPS, et al. Prosopis juliflora as a new cosmetic ingredient: Development and clinical evaluation of a bioactive moisturizing and anti-aging innovative solid core. Carbohydrate Polymers. 2020;**233**:115854

[41] Halla N, Heleno SA, Costa P, et al. Chemical profile and bioactive properties of the essential oil isolated from Ammodaucus leucotrichus fruits growing in Sahara and its evaluation as a cosmeceutical ingredient. Industrial Crops and Products. 2018;**119**:249-254

[42] Oargă DP, Cornea-Cipcigan M, Cordea MI. Unveiling the mechanisms for the development of rosehip-based dermatological products: An updated review. Frontiers in Pharmacology. 2024;**15**:1390419

[43] Desam NR, Al-Rajab AJ. The importance of natural products in cosmetics. In: Bioactive Natural Products for Pharmaceutical Applications. Berlin/Heidelberg, Germany: Springer; 2021. pp. 643-685

[44] Asche G. "80% of technical information found only in patents"–is there proof of this? World Patent Information. 2017;**48**:16-28

[45] Abe-Inge V, Aidoo R, de la Fuente MM, et al. Plant-based dietary

shift: Current trends, barriers, and carriers. Trends in Food Science and Technology. 2024;**143**:104292

[46] Fuentes JL, Pedraza Barrera CA, Villamizar Mantilla DA, et al. Flower extracts from ornamental plants as sources of sunscreen ingredients: Determination by in vitro methods of photoprotective efficacy, antigenotoxicity and safety. Molecules. 2022;**27**(17):5525

[47] Jiang B, Peng C, Li X, et al. Banana starch nanoparticles disrupt the integrity of the intestinal barrier by opening tight junctions in mice. Small. 2024;**24**(5):2408298

[48] Biskanaki F, Tertipi N, Andreou E, et al. The risk of using cosmetics and cosmetic procedures during pregnancy. Applied Sciences. 2024;**14**(21):9885

[49] Steinmetz FP, Wakefield JC, Boughton RM. Fractions of concern: Challenges and strategies for the safety assessment of biological matter in cosmetics. Cosmetics. 2021;**8**(2):34

Chapter 5

Are Sunscreens Safe?

Metin Özaslan

Abstract

Ultraviolet (UV) light is one of the main environmental factors that can lead to skin cancers, photoaging, and DNA mutations. Sunscreens can contain organic, inorganic, and naturally derived filters that absorb or reflect UV rays. Recently, concerns have been raised over the safety of sunscreen ingredients. However, the systemic absorption and long-term safety of these ingredients remain controversial. The FDA has reported that some organic filters enter the bloodstream and may have potential endocrine-disrupting effects. In particular, oxybenzone and octinoxate are banned in some regions due to hormonal dysfunction and environmental toxicity. Octocrylene has been found to produce benzophenone over time and has potential toxic effects. While available data support the benefits of sunscreens, there is a lack of long-term safety studies. More comprehensive toxicological analyses and regulatory standards are needed to assess the effects of sunscreens on both human health and the environment.

Keywords: critical wavelength, photoprotection, skin cancer, sunscreening agents, sunscreen application

1. Introduction

Sunlight reaching the Earth's surface consists of ultraviolet (UV) radiation, infrared radiation, and visible light, with the UV spectrum being the most significant. It is estimated that UV radiation is responsible for approximately 90% of skin cancers. Additionally, UV radiation can lead to both acute skin changes, such as erythema and sunburn, and chronic effects, including photoaging. Among the UV rays, UVC (100–280 nm) is absorbed by the atmosphere and does not reach the Earth's surface. UVB (280–315 nm) cannot penetrate beyond the epidermis, the outer layer of the skin, while UVA1 (300–400 nm) and UVA2 (315–340 nm) can penetrate the epidermis and reach the deeper dermis. UVB radiation, which is absorbed in the epidermis, is the primary cause of sunburn and tanning, whereas UVA radiation is mainly responsible for photoaging and skin carcinogenesis by damaging collagen and elastic fibers in the dermis. UV radiation is believed to induce DNA mutations through oxidative damage by generating free radicals in the skin. The use of sunscreen plays a crucial role in protecting against the harmful effects of UV radiation [1, 2]. In this chapter, we aim to explore the history of sunscreens, their ingredients, mechanisms of action, proper usage, and safety concerns.

2. A brief history of sunscreens

Throughout history, light skin has been regarded as a symbol of high cultural and social status. In Japan during the 700 s, people applied powder to their faces to achieve a white complexion, which was considered a mark of beauty. Similarly, in 1600s Europe, women used face-whitening cosmetics or velvet masks to prevent their light skin from darkening. In ancient Egyptian and Greek cultures, various natural substances, including rice bran, jasmine, olive oil, and lupine, were used for sun protection [3]. UV radiation was first discovered by Johann Wilhelm Ritter in 1801. In the early twentieth century, it became clear that UV rays were responsible for sunburn and tanning, prompting the development of sunscreens designed to block UVB rays. In 1969, Albert Kligman identified the phenomenon of photoaging, which led to the creation of sunscreens that filter UVA rays. The first UVB filters were benzyl salicylate and benzyl cinnamate, while the first UVA filter was avobenzone. In the latter half of the twentieth century, Rudolf Schulze worked on standardizing sun protection measurements, and in 1978, Franz Greiter introduced the Sun Protection Factor (SPF) as we know it today [4].

3. Sunscreens

3.1 Ingredients

An ideal sunscreen should effectively block the harmful effects of the sun by absorbing UV rays while maintaining stability. Degradation of the active molecules can result in reduced efficacy and potential toxicity. Additionally, it should be water-resistant, safe at low concentrations, inert, and nonirritating to the skin. Sunscreens are available in the market that contains organic, inorganic, and naturally derived UV filters. Organic filters in topical sunscreens absorb UV light, while inorganic filters reflect UV rays away from the skin. Although a combination of organic and inorganic filters is commonly used in sunscreen formulations, this may lead to catalytic processes that degrade their structure, ultimately reducing their effectiveness [5].

Naturally derived UV filters work through various mechanisms, such as UV absorption, inhibition of elastase and collagenase, and the elimination of free oxygen radicals. Examples of these filters include rosmarinic acid, carotenoids, raspberry and blueberry extracts, silymarin, lignin, and quercetin [4, 6]. The effectiveness and durability of sunscreen ingredients can vary depending on an individual's skin type and environmental conditions, which has led to the need for using multiple filters together. Furthermore, a sunscreen filter approved in one country may be considered hazardous in another. For instance, while Tinosorb, a broad-spectrum filter, is widely used in Europe, it is not approved by the FDA. Similarly, avobenzone and octinoxate are banned in Hawaii due to their environmental risks to coral reefs [7]. As a result, sunscreens with different ingredient combinations tailored to specific countries or regions have been introduced to the market (**Table 1**) [4, 6].

3.2 Basic terminology of sunscreens

Minimal erythema dose: The minimum radiation dose required to induce detectable erythema [8–10].

Type	Names	Effective UV spectrum	Organizations that have authorized	Highest allowable concentration
Organic	Avobenzone (Butyl methoxy-dibenzoylmethane)	UVA	FDA, ECHA, NMPA, TGA	3% (FDA), 5% (ECHA, TGA, NMPA)
	Aminobenzoic acid (Para-amino benzoic acid)	UVB	FDA, TGA	15%
	Bemotrizinol (Tinosorb S)	UVA, UVB	ECHA, TGA	10%
	Bisoctrizole (Tinosorb M)	UVA, UVB	ECHA, NMPA, TGA	10%
	Cinoxate	UVB	FDA, TGA	3% (FDA), 6% (TGA)
	Enzacamene (4-Methylbenzylidene Camphor)	UVA, UVB	ECHA, NMPA, TGA	4%
	Homosalate (Homomethyl salicylate)	UVB	ECHA, FDA, NMPA, TGA	15% (FDA), 10% (ECHA, NMPA, TGA)
	Meradimate (Menthyl anthranilate)	UVA, UVB	FDA, TGA	5%
	Mexoryl SL (Benzylidene camphor sulfonic acid)	UVB	ECHA, NMPA, TGA	6%
	Mexoryl SX (Ecamsule)	UVA, UVB	ECHA, NMPA, TGA	10%
	Mexoryl XL (DromeTRIzole trisiloxane)	UVA, UVB	ECHA, NMPA, TGA	10% (TGA), 15% (ECHA, NMPA)
	Mexoryl 400 (Methoxypropylamino cyclohexenylideneeth oxyethylcyanoacetate)	UVA	ECHA	3%
	NeoHeliopanAP (Bisdisulizole disodium)	UVA	ECHA, NMPA, TGA	10%
	Octinoxate (octyl methoxycinnamate)	UVB	ECHA, FDA, NMPA, TGA	7.5% (FDA), 10% (ECHA, NMPA, TGA)
	Octisalate (octylsalicylate)	UVB	ECHA, FDA, NMPA, TGA	5%
	Octocrylene (Uvinul N539)	UVB	ECHA, FDA, NMPA, TGA	10%
	Oxybenzone (Benzophenone-3)	UVA	ECHA, FDA, NMPA, TGA	6% (ECHA, FDA), 10%(NMPA, TGA)
	Padimate O (Ethylhexyl dimethyl PABA)	UVB	FDA, HC, NMPA	8%

Type	Names	Effective UV spectrum	Organizations that have authorized	Highest allowable concentration
	Piperazine	UVA	ECHA	
	Uvinul T150 (Ethylhexyl triazone)	UVB	ECHA, NMPA, TGA	5%
Inorganic	Titanium dioxide (TiO_2)	UVA, UVB	ECHA, FDA, NMPA, TGA	25%
	Tris-biphenyl triazine (TBPT)	UVB	ECHA, TGA	10%
	Trolamine salicylate (Aspergel)	UVB	FDA, TGA	12%
	Zinc oxide (ZnO)	UVA, UVB	ECHA, FDA, NMPA, TGA	25% (ECHA, FDA, NMPA), No Limit (TGA)

ECHA: European Chemicals Agency, FDA: U.S Food and Drug Administration, NMPA: National Medical Products Administration, TGA: Therapeutics Good Administration.

Table 1.
Organic and inorganic UV filters.

Sun/sunburn protection factor (SPF): Ratio between the minimal erythemal doses (MED) of skin protected by sunscreen application of 2 mg/cm^2 and unprotected skin.

UVA protection factor (UVAPF): Ratio of the UV-A dose required for minimum darkening on protected skin to the UV-A dose required for the same effect on unprotected skin.

Immune protection factor (IPF): The capability of sunscreens to prevent UV-induced immunosuppression.

Critical wavelength: The wavelength at which 90% of the UV absorption of sunscreen occurs.

Broad-spectrum sunscreen: Sunscreen with critical wavelength > 370 nm and UVA protection factor > 4.

Water-resistant sunscreen: After two consecutive immersions in water for 20 minutes (a total of 40 minutes), the product retains its SPF value.

Very water-resistant sunscreen: After two consecutive immersions in water for 20 minutes (a total of 80 minutes), the product retains its SPF value.

3.3 Regulatory requirements in the USA and Europe

In various countries, different criteria have been established to ensure that sunscreens meet minimum qualification standards. In the United States, the FDA-defined method is used to measure *in vitro* UV transmittance through sunscreen film. Known as the critical wavelength method, this approach requires that UVB-filtering sunscreens have a minimum critical wavelength of 320 nm, while broad-spectrum UVA and UVB-filtering sunscreens must have a minimum critical wavelength of 370 nm. In the United Kingdom, the Boots Star Rating System is employed. This system measures UV absorption between 290 and 400 nm by reflecting UV light onto polymethyl methacrylate plates, with the rating based on the average UVA/UVB ratio. Sunscreens with a ratio of 0.6 or above can receive a star rating, and a ratio of 0.9 or above earns a five-star rating, offering more protection than sunscreen with a ratio between 0.6 and 0.79 (three stars). In European countries, the COLIPA method is used. COLIPA is an association that sets standards for the labeling and testing of sunscreens in the cosmetics industry [11]. European guidelines require that sunscreens have a UVAPF value, measured by persistent pigment darkening (PPD) (*in vivo*) or COLIPA (*in vitro*), of at least one-third of the SPF *in vivo* value, along with protection against the minimum critical wavelength of 370 nm. Sunscreens available in the market are categorized by SPF values, including SPF 50+ (very high), SPF 30 or 50 (high), SPF 15, 20, or 25 (medium), and SPF 6 or 10 (low protection) [12].

Japan and Australia have established their own standards for UV protection factors. In Australia, UVA protection is defined by a sunscreen product's ability to transmit less than 10% of light between 320 and 360 nm through an 8 μm layer of the product. In Japan, the UVAPF is calculated as the ratio of the minimal permanent pigment darkening (MPPD) dose of protected skin to the MPPD dose of unprotected skin. According to this system, if the UVAPF value of a product is between 2 and 4, it provides low protection; if it is between 4 and 8, it offers medium protection; and if it is greater than 8, it provides high protection [12].

3.4 Sunscreen application method

The American Academy of Dermatology recommends using sunscreens with at least SPF30, with SPF50 being considered ideal for optimal protection. For effective sun protection, it is advised that all sun-exposed areas be covered with sunscreen at a thickness of 2 mg/cm^2 (about one ounce). However, as the SPF of a sunscreen increases, the level of UV protection does not rise proportionally. For instance, SPF15 provides 93.3% protection, SPF30 offers 96.7% protection, and SPF50 provides 98% protection. Despite these recommendations, studies show that 30–50% of consumers fail to apply the optimal amount of sunscreen, leading to a significant decrease in its effectiveness. For example, applying only 1 mg/cm^2 of an SPF50 sunscreen, instead of the recommended 2 mg/cm^2, results in an SPF effect of just 26 [13, 14].

It is essential to reapply sunscreen every 2 hours, regardless of environmental conditions such as snow, clouds, or rain, as well as after sweating or water exposure, to maintain its effectiveness. The choice of sunscreen formulation should be based on skin type and the area of application. Creams are ideal for dry skin, gels work well for hairy areas, sticks are suitable for the eye area and lips, and sprays are recommended for children. For infants under 6 months of age, sun protection methods such as hats and long-sleeved clothing are generally preferred over the use of sunscreen [14].

3.5 Safety concerns regarding sunscreens

In the United States, sunscreens are regulated as medicines, rather than cosmetics, which requires FDA approval. In 1999, the FDA-approved 16 UV filters, with ecamsule being the only addition since then. In 2019, the FDA categorized sunscreen ingredients into three groups based on their safety profiles. Ingredients classified as Generally Recognized as Safe and Effective (GRASE) are supported by clinical data showing no carcinogenic or reproductive risks. Ingredients deemed not safe and effective are placed in Category 2, while those requiring further data to assess their safety are classified as Category 3 (**Table 2**) [15].

In addition to the well-known and relatively minor side effects of sunscreens, such as contact dermatitis and clothing staining, recent studies suggest that they may also contribute to hormonal dysfunction, as well as reproductive and neurological system toxicities [16]. The FDA confirmed systemic absorption of organic sunscreen filters in two studies published in 2019 and 2020. These studies showed that blood levels of active ingredients exceeded the FDA's threshold of 0.5 ng/mL after repeated applications of organic sunscreens at a concentration of 2 mg/cm^2 on 75% of the body

Grase	Not Grase	Further data needed
Titanium dioxide	Aminobenzoic acid	Avobenzone
Zinc oxide	Trolamine salicylate	Cinoxate
		Dioxybenzone
		Ensulizole
		Homosalate
		Meradimate
		Octinoxate
		Octisalate
		Octocrylene
		Oxybenzone
		Padimate O
		Sulisobenzone

GRASE: Generally Recognized as Safe and Effective.

Table 2.
Classification of UV filters according to safety categories.

surface [17, 18]. Although these findings do not indicate clinically harmful effects, the demonstration of systemic absorption highlights the need for long-term safety data on sunscreens. Furthermore, the FDA's safety threshold of 0.5 ng/mL may not detect high absorption in some cases, and low absorption rates could lead to potential risks being overlooked. Long-term use of sunscreens may result in accumulation in the body, thereby increasing the risk of toxicity. This threshold may also be insufficient for vulnerable groups such as children, the elderly, and pregnant women. As a result, more sensitive testing methods and comprehensive toxicological assessments may be necessary to ensure the safety of sunscreens [19].

3.5.1 Oxybenzone and octinoxate

In 2018 and 2019, Hawaii and Key West banned sunscreens containing oxybenzone (benzophenone-3) and octinoxate (octyl methoxycinnamate) due to their toxicity to marine ecosystems. These ingredients have the potential to disrupt endocrine function and can enter the body through the skin, as well as being found in air, water, cosmetics, and plastics, in addition to sunscreens. These substances have been detected in various body fluids, including urine, blood, and breast milk. However, their impact on human health remains unclear [20].

The effects of oxybenzone on thyroid hormones, reproductive hormones, kidney function, and fetal development have been studied. The general consensus regarding prenatal exposure to oxybenzone is that there is no significant association with sex ratio, birth weight, or IQ. Although animal studies have shown that oxybenzone can affect thyroid hormones, these results are inconsistent in human studies [20]. In a study involving 32 individuals in which sunscreen containing 10% concentration of oxybenzone was applied daily to the whole body, it was shown that serum thyroid hormone levels were not affected at week 1 compared to baseline [21].

A recent meta-analysis concluded that oxybenzone (at a concentration of 1 μM) acts as a thyroid receptor agonist, but does not alter thyroid hormone synthesis or thyroid peroxidase activity. Benzophenone-1 (BP-1), a metabolite of oxybenzone, was found to activate thyroid peroxidase at a very low concentration (0.001 μM) in human follicular thyroid cells and at a high concentration (32 μM) altered thyroid hormone gene expression in rats [22]. Further studies are needed to clarify the potential effects of oxybenzone and BP-1 on thyroid function.

Oxybenzone has estrogenic and anti-androgenic activities. Its effects on the reproductive system include decreased human sperm motility (EC50: 4.7 μM), inhibition of oocyte maturation in mice (at a concentration of 0.5 μM), negative effects on follicle population, impaired placental development, disrupted milk protein synthesis, and altered mammary gland differentiation. BP-1 may exert anti-androgenic effects by inhibiting the enzyme responsible for converting androstenedione, a precursor to testosterone, into testosterone [22].

Concerning renal function, a study conducted with 441 healthy young women examined the urinary albumin-creatinine ratio after oxybenzone exposure and found an association with an impaired albumin-creatinine ratio, which may indicate kidney damage [23].

Oxybenzone has been recognized as "Contact Allergen of the Year" by The North American Contact Dermatitis Group, as it is one of the most common agents causing contact dermatitis among sunscreens. Benzophenone-1 has the potential to cause phototoxic effects by increasing free radical production in keratinocytes. The presence of oxybenzone in the blood, placenta, and amniotic fluid has raised concerns about its potential adverse effects on fetal development, though these effects are generally considered minimal. Despite data suggesting that oxybenzone may increase DNA hypomethylation and susceptibility to neurodegenerative diseases in mice, there is no evidence of neurotoxic effects in humans [24].

Long-term exposure to octinoxate (octyl methoxycinnamate) has been associated with various adverse health effects, including hypothyroidism, changes in puberty, asthma, and breast cancer. An *in vitro* study on human umbilical artery cells suggested that long-term exposure to octinoxate may be linked to hypertensive disorders in pregnancy. It is recommended to avoid octinoxate for children, adolescents, and pregnant women. Further long-term studies on its toxicity are needed to clarify the risk-benefit balance of octinoxate [25, 26].

3.5.2 Octocrylene (uvinul N539)

Octocrylene is one of the most widely used UV filters. Both *in vitro* and *in vivo* studies show that octocrylene has limited absorption through the skin and results in low systemic circulation levels. Toxicological data suggest that octocrylene does not have endocrine-disrupting effects and does not pose any adverse effects on reproductive or developmental parameters. Skin irritation is rare, and the risk of photoallergic reactions is increased, particularly in individuals with a history of topical ketoprofen use [27]. However, it has been found that benzophenone levels in sunscreen products containing octocrylene increase over time. Benzophenone is a byproduct of the retro-aldol reaction of octocrylene. Benzophenone is known to be a mutagen, carcinogen, and hormonal disruptor. It is banned in the United States for use in food products and packaging, and there is no established safe limit for its presence in personal care products [28].

In another study, octocrylene was linked to obesity by increasing adiponectin production during adipogenesis in stem cells, exhibiting a partial agonist effect on PPARγ, and altering lipid metabolism gene expression in human keratinocytes [29].

3.5.3 Uvinul 400 (benzophenon-1)

Benzophenone-1 (BP-1) is a chemical commonly used in sunscreens and cosmetics, primarily entering the human body through dermal absorption. It can also be detected in drinking water, seafood, and packaged foods. BP-1 has been associated with skin irritation and allergic reactions. Furthermore, it can induce oxidative stress in the nervous system, potentially contributing to cognitive impairments, including memory and learning disorders, and has been linked to neurodegenerative diseases such as Alzheimer's and Parkinson's. Additionally, BP-1 exposure may result in DNA damage and chromosomal abnormalities, and can negatively impact liver and kidney function [30]. BP-1 has estrogenic and anti-androgenic effects; these effects have been associated with testicular cancer and ovarian cancer metastasis [30–32]. These effects have been predominantly demonstrated *in vitro* or in animal studies. A review examining human exposure to benzophenones reported that BP-1 was detected in approximately 20% of semen samples from men, suggesting a potential negative impact on male fertility. In women, a possible association between BP-1 exposure and the development of endometriosis was also discussed [33]. Given these potentially harmful effects, further research is needed to minimize BP-1 exposure and better understand its health effects.

3.5.4 Homosalate (homomethyl salicylate)

Due to its lipophilic nature, homosalate has been reported to strongly bind to skin layers and can be absorbed into the systemic circulation following topical application. Data on its genotoxic effects are limited; however, it may induce DNA damage in human lymphocytes. It is also suggested that homosalate could cause DNA damage through the generation of free oxygen radicals [34].

Studies investigating the potential biological effects of homosalate have shown that it can exhibit both agonistic and antagonistic activities by binding to human estrogen receptor alpha and androgen receptors. Its estrogenic activity has been reported to promote the proliferation of breast cancer cells. However, comprehensive data on the long-term effects of homosalate on human health, particularly concerning reproductive and developmental processes, remain limited [35]. Research on the effects of homosalate on thyroid function is limited. *In vitro* studies have demonstrated that high doses of homosalate induce genotoxic effects in rat thyroid cells, but not in human thyroid cells. Additionally, homosalate was found to increase the expression of both thyroglobulin (TG) and thyroid peroxidase (TPO) genes in rat cells, while only upregulating the TG gene in human cells. The clinical relevance of these findings regarding the impact of homosalate on thyroid function remains unclear [36].

3.5.5 Padimate O (ethylhexyl dimethyl PABA)

PABA was one of the first sunscreen ingredients to be widely used. However, its use has declined over time due to the requirement for an alcohol-based carrier, the tendency to stain clothing, and its potential to cause skin irritation and allergic reactions. Padimate O, an ester derivative of PABA, has been identified as the most effective FDA-approved UVB filter. It has gained greater popularity than PABA due to its improved compatibility with cosmetic formulations and reduced tendency to cause staining [37]. However, Padimate O has raised safety concerns due to its potential genotoxic effects. *In vitro*, studies have demonstrated that skin cells exposed to sunscreens containing Padimate O can experience indirect DNA damage, such as strand breaks, when subjected to UV light [38]. Another *in vitro* study showed that Padimate O can induce DNA damage by generating reactive oxygen species upon irradiation, particularly affecting GC base pairs [39].

3.5.6 Enzacamane (4- methylbenzylidene camphor)

Enzacamene is a UV filter commonly used in cosmetic products. Even at low doses, it can accumulate in the body and exert systemic effects. It has been shown to increase the production of proinflammatory molecules, such as TNF-α and IL-6, and to interfere with DNA repair mechanisms. Due to its endocrine-disrupting properties, enzacamene may negatively impact on reproductive health. Estrogenic and anti-androgenic effects have been observed in mice, and *in vitro* studies have demonstrated its ability to bind to the human estrogen receptor beta, suggesting potential estrogenic activity [40, 41].

In addition to its effects on reproductive health, enzacamene may impair embryo implantation and the sperm acrosome reaction. However, most of these effects have been observed in cell cultures, and it remains unclear how they would manifest in actual human exposure. While the concentrations of enzacamene measured in humans are at levels that could potentially cause effects in animal models, the precise risks to human health are not yet fully understood. Further research is needed to better assess the long-term effects of enzacamene and its accumulation in the body [42].

3.5.7 Titanium dioxide (TiO_2) ve zinc oxide (ZnO)

Among the potential risks of titanium dioxide and zinc oxide filters, health concerns related to inhalation exposure are particularly notable. Inhalation of products in spray or powder form may lead to the accumulation of nanoparticles in the lungs. The respirable form of TiO2 is classified as a potential carcinogen by the International Agency for Research on Cancer (IARC). As a result, cream or lotion formulations of these filters are considered safer. Additionally, unlike organic UV filters, there is no scientific evidence linking titanium dioxide or zinc oxide to hormonal disruptions. The risk of irritant and allergic reactions, which are common with organic filters, is also much lower with inorganic filters. Environmentally, they are a more eco-friendly alternative, as their negative impact on coral reefs and aquatic ecosystems is less significant compared to that of organic filters [43].

3.6 Environmental concerns about sunscreens

Organic UV filters are also widely used as photostabilizers in products beyond sunscreens, including fragrances, shampoos, personal cosmetics, and plastics. The Centers for Disease Control and Prevention (CDC) has suggested that 97% of the U.S. population has been exposed to oxybenzone. These UV filters have been commonly detected in water supplies, particularly oxybenzone. Organic filters are absorbed through the skin and are subsequently released into the environment *via* urine or during showering. UV filters, such as octinoxate and octocrylene, have been found in higher concentrations in densely populated areas, especially during the summer. In swimming pools, these filters can react with chlorine, forming toxic by-products, with chlorinated oxybenzone leading to an increased rate of cell death [44]. Wastewater treatment plants are also ineffective at removing UV filters due to their low water solubility and highly lipophilic nature, resulting in these chemicals being returned to the water supply. Approximately 4% of oxybenzone is absorbed through the skin, while the remaining 96% is washed away and ends up in water sources. It is estimated that 8000–16,000 tons of sunscreen are released into coral reefs each year. Oxybenzone can cause coral bleaching, coral death, and toxic effects on larvae, even at low concentrations. Additionally, it accumulates in fish, leading to reproductive issues and hormonal imbalances, which negatively impact the entire ecosystem [45].

Exposure of crucian carp to dibenzoyl methane derivatives and Padimate O (concentrations ranging from 3.88 to 337.15 μg/L) has been shown to induce neurotoxicity and oxidative stress in the liver. When the toxicity of UV filter mixtures was assessed, both antagonistic and synergistic effects were observed. A mixture of oxybenzone, octinoxate, and enzacamene (concentrations between 0.1 and 100 mg/L) reduced mortality in *Chironomus riparius* compared to exposure to a single UV filter, indicating that these substances attenuated each other's effects. In contrast, the combination of oxybenzone and enzacamene demonstrated a synergistic effect, enhancing the expression of the hsp70 gene compared to individual exposure [46].

UV filters with a high oil/water distribution coefficient (log pow ≥ 4.5) are considered to have a greater potential for bioaccumulation (**Table 3**) [47].

UV filter	Log pow	Bioaccumulation risk
Bis-Ethylhexyloxyphenol Methoxyphenyl Triazine	>5.7	High
Diethylamino Hydroxybenzoyl Hexyl Benzoate	6.2	
Ethylhexyl Triazone	≥7	
Avobenzone	6.1	
Padimate O	>6.2	
Octinoxate	>6	
Octisalate	5.94	
Homosalate	6.27	
Polysilicone-15	5.66	
Octocrylene	6.1	
Tris-Biphenyl Triazine	>5.6	
Phenylene Bis-Diphenyltriazine	10.5	Very high
Bisoctrizole	12.7	

Table 3.
Classification of UV filters according to bioaccumulation risk.

The effects of UV filters on soil and sediment ecosystems remain unclear. Most research has focused on aquatic organisms, while the impact on terrestrial microorganisms, insects, and plants has not been sufficiently studied [47]. There is evidence of bioaccumulation in land animals, particularly birds. In a Spanish study, several UV filters were detected in the eggs of various bird species. It is suggested that the mothers were exposed to these filters through contaminated water sources and subsequently transferred them to their eggs [48].

4. Conclusions

Chronic exposure to sunlight can lead to serious health issues, such as skin cancer and photoaging. Therefore, the use of sunscreens is important, but their potential harms have also become the focus of recent research.

There is limited data on the effects of organic sunscreens on human health. Evidence suggests possible harm to the hormonal and reproductive systems from oxybenzone and octinoxate, mutagenic effects of octocrylene by increasing benzophenone levels, and potential adverse effects of uvinul 400 on fertility. However, the exact dosages and durations required for these effects to manifest are not yet clearly understood.

The environmental impact of UV filters has been particularly studied in aquatic ecosystems, where it has been shown that some components negatively affect fish health and can cause coral bleaching. Nevertheless, climate change is widely recognized as the primary threat to coral reefs. Additionally, the long-term human health and environmental effects of many new UV filters are still not fully known.

Considering the available scientific data, the health risks associated with not using sunscreen outweigh the potential side effects. For those concerned about organic UV filters, products containing inorganic filters like ZnO and TiO_2 may offer a reliable alternative.

Further research on the safety of sunscreens is essential. Manufacturers, healthcare professionals, environmental scientists, and regulatory bodies must collaborate to address concerns regarding the reliability of these products. Doctors should stay updated with current scientific data to educate the public and provide guidance on the proper use of sunscreens. It is crucial for individuals to be informed about the types of sunscreens and effective application methods, as this plays a key role in protecting skin health.

Author details

Metin Özaslan
Konya Numune Hospital, Konya, Turkey

*Address all correspondence to: metinozaslanx@gmail.com

References

[1] Serpone N. Sunscreens and their usefulness: Have we made any progress in the last two decades? Photochemical and Photobiological Sciences. 2021;**20**(2):189-244

[2] Sander M, Sander M, Burbidge T, Beecker J. The efficacy and safety of sunscreen use for the prevention of skin cancer. Canadian Medical Association Journal. 2020;**192**(50):E1802-E1808. Available from: http://www.cmaj.ca/lookup/doi/10.1503/cmaj.201085

[3] Drissi M, Carr E, Housewright C. Sunscreen: A brief walk through history. Baylor University Medical Center Proceedings. 2022;**35**(1):121-123

[4] Salih H, Psomadakis C, George SMC. Sunscreens: A narrative review. Skin Health and Disease. 2024;**4**(6):e432. Available from: https://academic.oup.com/skinhd/article/doi/10.1002/ski2.432/7950880

[5] Mewada R, Shah Y. Recent advances in sunscreen agents and their formulations: A review. International Journal of Pharmaceutical Chemistry and Analysis. 2023;**9**(4):141-150

[6] Chavda VP, Acharya D, Hala V, Daware S, Vora LK. Sunscreens: A comprehensive review with the application of nanotechnology. Journal of Drug Delivery Science and Technology. 2023;**86**:104720. Available from: https://linkinghub.elsevier.com/retrieve/pii/S1773224723005725

[7] Van HT. Uses and mechanism of action of main ingredients in sunscreen products. Middle East Journal of Applied Science and Technology. 2024;**07**(02):108-116

[8] Schalka S, dos Reis VMS. Fator de proteção solar: significado e controvérsias. Anais Brasileiros de Dermatologia. 2011;**86**(3):507-515. Available from: http://www.scielo.br/scielo.php?script=sci_arttext&pid=S0365-05962011000300013&lng=pt&tlng=pt

[9] Kaimal S, Abraham A. Sunscreens. Indian Journal of Dermatology, Venereology and Leprology. 2011;**77**(2):238-243

[10] Césarini J, Christiaens F, Cole C, Herzog B, Hönigsmann H, Osterwalder U, et al. UVA Protection and Sunscreens. Vienna, Austria: Commission Internationale de l'Éclairage (CIE); 2010. Available from: http://www.cie.co.at/

[11] Donglikar MM, Deore SL. Sunscreens: A review. Pharmacognosy Journal. 2016;**8**(3):171-179

[12] Latha M, Martis J, Sham Shinde R, Bangera S, Krishnankutty B, Bellary S, et al. Sunscreening agents a review. The Journal of Clinical and Aesthetic Dermatology. 2013;**6**(1):16-26

[13] Bennett SL, Khachemoune A. Dispelling myths about sunscreen. Journal of Dermatological Treatment. 2022;**33**(2):666-670. Available from: https://www.tandfonline.com/doi/full/10.1080/09546634.2020.1789047

[14] Ida O, Usman A, Leila E. Sun protection: A comprehensive 2022 dermatologic review. Journal of Family Medicine and Disease Prevention. 2023;**9**(1):154. Available from: https://clinmedjournals.org/articles/jfmdp/journal-of-family-medicine-and-disease-prevention-jfmdp-9-154.php?jid=jfmdp

[15] Abdel Azim S, Bainvoll L, Vecerek N, DeLeo VA, Adler BL. Sunscreens part 2: Regulation and safety. Journal of the American Academy of Dermatology. 2024:S0190-9622(24)00786-2

[16] Adler BL. Sunscreen safety: 2024 updates. Cutis. 2024;**113**(5):195-196

[17] Matta MK, Zusterzeel R, Pilli NR, Patel V, Volpe DA, Florian J, et al. Effect of sunscreen application under maximal use conditions on plasma concentration of sunscreen active ingredients. Journal of the American Medical Association. 2019;**321**(21):2082

[18] Matta MK, Florian J, Zusterzeel R, Pilli NR, Patel V, Volpe DA, et al. Effect of sunscreen application on plasma concentration of sunscreen active ingredients. Journal of the American Medical Association. 2020;**323**(3):256

[19] Wang J, Ganley CJ. Safety threshold considerations for sunscreen systemic exposure: A simulation study. Clinical Pharmacology and Therapeutics. 2019;**105**(1):161-167

[20] Suh S, Pham C, Smith J, Mesinkovska NA. The banned sunscreen ingredients and their impact on human health: A systematic review. International Journal of Dermatology. 2020;**59**(9):1033-1042

[21] Janjua NR, Kongshoj B, Petersen JH, Wulf HC. Sunscreens and thyroid function in humans after short-term whole-body topical application: A single-blinded study. British Journal of Dermatology. 2007;**156**(5):1080-1082. Available from: https://academic.oup.com/bjd/article/156/5/1080/6640827

[22] Mustieles V, Balogh RK, Axelstad M, Montazeri P, Márquez S, Vrijheid M, et al. Benzophenone-3: Comprehensive review of the toxicological and human evidence with meta-analysis of human biomonitoring studies. Environment International. 2023;**173**:107739. Available from: https://linkinghub.elsevier.com/retrieve/pii/S0160412023000120

[23] Kang H, Kim S, Lee G, Lee I, Lee JP, Lee J, et al. Urinary metabolites of dibutyl phthalate and benzophenone-3 are potential chemical risk factors of chronic kidney function markers among healthy women. Environment International. 2019;**124**:354-360. Available from: https://linkinghub.elsevier.com/retrieve/pii/S0160412018330599

[24] Wnuk W, Michalska K, Krupa A, Pawlak K. Benzophenone-3, a chemical UV-filter in cosmetics: Is it really safe for children and pregnant women? Advances in Dermatology and Allergology. 2022;**39**(1):26-33. Available from: https://www.termedia.pl/doi/10.5114/ada.2022.113617

[25] Lorigo M, Quintaneiro C, Breitenfeld L, Cairrao E. Exposure to UV-B filter octylmethoxycinnamate and human health effects: Focus on endocrine disruptor actions. Chemosphere. 2024;**358**:142218

[26] Lorigo M, Quintaneiro C, Maia CJ, Breitenfeld L, Cairrao E. UV-B filter octylmethoxycinnamate impaired the main vasorelaxant mechanism of human umbilical artery. Chemosphere. 2021;**277**:130302. Available from: https://linkinghub.elsevier.com/retrieve/pii/S0045653521007724

[27] Berardesca E, Zuberbier T, Sanchez Viera M, Marinovich M. Review of the safety of octocrylene used as an ultraviolet filter in cosmetics. Journal of the European Academy of Dermatology and Venereology. 2019;**33**(S7):25-33

[28] Downs CA, Dinardo JC, Stien D, Rodrigues AMS, Lebaron P.

Benzophenone accumulates over time from the degradation of octocrylene in commercial sunscreen products. Chemical Research in Toxicology. 2021;**34**(4):1046-1054

[29] Ko H, An S, Ahn S, Park IG, Gong J, Hwang SY, et al. Sunscreen filter octocrylene is a potential obesogen by acting as a PPARγ partial agonist. Toxicology Letters. 2022;**355**:141-149

[30] Yao YN, Wang Y, Zhang H, Gao Y, Zhang T, Kannan K. A review of sources, pathways, and toxic effects of human exposure to benzophenone ultraviolet light filters. Eco-Environment and Health. 2024;**3**(1):30-44

[31] Nashev LG, Schuster D, Laggner C, Sodha S, Langer T, Wolber G, et al. The UV-filter benzophenone-1 inhibits 17β-hydroxysteroid dehydrogenase type 3: Virtual screening as a strategy to identify potential endocrine disrupting chemicals. Biochemical Pharmacology. 2010;**79**(8):1189-1199

[32] Shin S, Go RE, Kim CW, Hwang KA, Nam KH, Choi KC. Effect of benzophenone-1 and octylphenol on the regulation of epithelial-mesenchymal transition via an estrogen receptor-dependent pathway in estrogen receptor expressing ovarian cancer cells. Food and Chemical Toxicology. 2016;**93**:58-65

[33] Mao JF, Li W, Ong CN, He Y, Jong MC, Gin KYH. Assessment of human exposure to benzophenone-type UV filters: A review. Environment International. 2022;**167**:107405. Available from: https://linkinghub.elsevier.com/retrieve/pii/S0160412022003324

[34] Yazar S, Gökçek Y. Assessment of in vitro genotoxicity effect of homosalate in cosmetics. Marmara Pharmaceutical Journal. 2018;**22**(3):436-442

[35] Krause M, Klit A, Blomberg Jensen M, Søeborg T, Frederiksen H, Schlumpf M, et al. Sunscreens: Are they beneficial for health? An overview of endocrine disrupting properties of UV-filters. International Journal of Andrology. 2012;**35**(3):424-436

[36] Coperchini F, Greco A, Teliti M, Denegri M, Croce L, Calì B, et al. In vitro study of the UV-filter homosalate effects on rat and human thyroid cells. Environmental Pollution. 2024;**363**:125063. Available from: https://linkinghub.elsevier.com/retrieve/pii/S0269749124017809

[37] Levy SB. Sunscreens. In: Comprehensive Dermatologic Drug Therapy: Expert Consult - Online and Print. Philadelphia, PA, USA: Saunders (Elsevier); 2012. pp. 551-561.e1

[38] Gulston M, Knowland J. Illumination of human keratinocytes in the presence of the sunscreen ingredient padimate-O and through an SPF-15 sunscreen reduces direct photodamage to DNA but increases strand breaks. Mutation Research/Genetic Toxicology and Environmental Mutagenesis. 1999;**444**(1):49-60. Available from: https://linkinghub.elsevier.com/retrieve/pii/S1383571899000911

[39] McHugh PJ, Knowland J. Characterization of DNA damage inflicted by free radicals from a mutagenic sunscreen ingredient and its location using an in vitro genetic reversion assay. Photochemistry and Photobiology. 1997;**66**(2):276-281 Available from: https://onlinelibrary.wiley.com/doi/10.1111/j.1751-1097.1997.tb08655.x

[40] Schlumpf M, Schmid P, Durrer S, Conscience M, Maerkel K, Henseler M, et al. Endocrine activity and developmental toxicity of cosmetic

UV filters - An update. Toxicology. 2004;**205**(1-2 SPEC. ISS):113-122

[41] Schlumpf M, Jarry H, Wuttke W, Ma R, Lichtensteiger W. Estrogenic activity and estrogen receptor β binding of the UV filter 3-benzylidene camphor: Comparison with 4-methylbenzylidene camphor. Toxicology. 2004;**199**(2-3):109-120

[42] Lax C, Wicksell E, Grip A, Niemi JVL, Liu W, Rafeletou A, et al. The effect of sunscreen 4-methylbenzylidene camphor in different and reproductive models, its bioaccumulation and molecular effects on ligand-receptor interaction, and protein expression. Basic and Clinical Pharmacology and Toxicology. 2023;**133**(2):130-141

[43] Schneider SL, Lim HW. A review of inorganic UV filters zinc oxide and titanium dioxide. Photodermatology, Photoimmunology and Photomedicine. 2019;**35**(6):442-446

[44] Schneider SL, Lim HW. Review of environmental effects of oxybenzone and other sunscreen active ingredients. Journal of the American Academy of Dermatology. 2019;**80**(1):266-271

[45] DiNardo JC, Downs CA. Dermatological and environmental toxicological impact of the sunscreen ingredient oxybenzone/benzophenone-3. Journal of Cosmetic Dermatology. 2018;**17**(1):15-19

[46] Huang Y, Law JCF, Lam TK, Leung KSY. Risks of organic UV filters: A review of environmental and human health concern studies. Science of the Total Environment. 2021;**755**:142486

[47] Pawlowski S, Luetjens LH, Preibisch A, Acker S, Petersen-Thiery M. Cosmetic UV filters in the environment—State of the art in EU regulations, science and possible knowledge gaps. International Journal of Cosmetic Science. 2023;**45**(S1):52-66

[48] Couselo-Rodríguez C, González-Esteban PC, Diéguez Montes MP, Flórez Á. Impacto de los filtros ultravioleta en el entorno natural. Actas Dermo-Sifiliográficas. 2022;**113**(8):792-803

Chapter 6

Plant-Based Sunscreens: Innovations and New Formulations

Cristina Lungu, Adina Catinca Grădinaru and Bianca Ivănescu

Abstract

This book chapter corresponds with the modern trends that aim to include natural plant compounds and vegetal extracts in dermocosmetics and cosmeceuticals. Today, there is an increased tendency to obtain new cosmetic formulations that are eco-friendly, non-toxic, hypoallergenic, and possess antioxidant and anti-inflammatory effects. In this perspective, the main purpose of this chapter is to review the applications and limitations of some natural compounds and vegetal extracts (*Aloe vera, Mauritia flexuosa, Elaeagnus angustifolia, Punica granatum, Daucus carota, Cocos nucifera,* and others) in skin photoprotection and to present the latest topical formulations based on plants developed to increase their effectiveness.

Keywords: sunscreen, UV radiation, natural compounds from plants, vegetal extracts, modern formulations

1. Introduction

Sun exposure plays a significant role in human health, offering both benefits and risks. Moderate sun exposure is the primary natural source of vitamin D synthesis, which is crucial for bone health and immune function. Sunlight increases melanogenesis, which acts as a natural sunscreen and has an anti-inflammatory effect in some cutaneous conditions such as acne, psoriasis, and eczema. It is also linked to improved mood and circadian rhythm regulation [1, 2]. However, the positive effects are outweighed by the risks associated with prolonged or unprotected exposure to ultraviolet (UV) radiation.

The sun emits three types of UV radiation: UVA (315–400 nm), UVB (280–315 nm), and UVC (100–280 nm). Although UVC radiation has the highest energy in the UV spectrum and is the most harmful to human DNA, inducing carcinogenesis, it is largely absorbed by the Earth's ozone layer and does not reach the surface [3]. About 90–99% of UVA and 1–10% of UVB rays reach the Earth's surface, having a substantial impact on skin and overall health [1]. UVB rays are only capable of reaching the epidermis and are primarily responsible for sunburns, as they damage the DNA in epidermal cells, triggering inflammation and redness. UVA rays are able to penetrate deep into the dermis and accelerate the breakdown of collagen and elastin fibers, leading to premature aging, wrinkles, and loss of skin elasticity. They cause photoaging, immunosuppression, and skin cancer [3]. Chronic exposure to both UVA and UVB radiation increases the risk of skin cancers, including basal cell carcinoma, squamous cell carcinoma, and the more aggressive melanoma. UV radiation causes DNA mutations, oxidative stress, and immune suppression, all of which contribute to carcinogenesis [4].

Overexposure can cause hyperpigmentation issues such as melasma and age spots and can damage the skin microbiome, reducing host immunity. UV rays can also harm the eyes, contributing to cataracts and macular degeneration. Excessive UV exposure may suppress the immune system, reducing the skin's ability to combat infections and increasing susceptibility to diseases. It can also exacerbate autoimmune conditions like lupus and increase oxidative stress in tissues, potentially accelerating aging and chronic disease development [2].

In recent years, other types of radiation with less energy, have been shown to possess deleterious effects on human health, such as blue light, near-infrared radiation, and long UVA. Near-infrared radiation is involved in photoaging along with UVA radiation [5]. Exposure to blue light from smartphones, computers, tablets, and electronic devices in general greatly contributes to extrinsic skin aging. Blue light penetrates up to 1 mm into the dermis and induces the formation of free radicals, resulting in DNA damage, hyperpigmentation, skin aging, and deregulation of the circadian rhythm [6].

To mitigate the harmful effects of UV radiation, sunscreens are formulated with UV filters that either absorb, reflect, or scatter harmful rays. UV filters are broadly classified into organic (chemical) and inorganic (physical) filters. Organic UV filters absorb UV radiation and convert it into heat through a photochemical reaction, preventing the rays from penetrating the skin. These filters are composed of aromatic compounds that contain conjugated double bonds, which allow them to absorb specific UV wavelengths. Since UVB causes immediate and serious sunburn, most organic UV filters protect against UVB rays, and only a few can protect against UVA rays [1]. Because each filter has a limited spectral band of absorption, in order to achieve broad-spectrum protection, they are mainly used in combination, with the maximum additive concentration ranging from 2 to 20% in the EU, USA, China, and Japan [7].

Inorganic filters, also known as mineral filters, act by reflecting and scattering UV radiation away from the skin. They are composed of non-toxic, naturally occurring minerals (zinc oxide, titanium dioxide) and are generally considered safer and more environmentally friendly. Inorganic filters offer broader coverage by blocking both UVB and UVA radiations and are more photostable. They are less likely to cause allergic reactions or irritation by penetrating only up to the dermis layer, making them ideal for sensitive skin types. The disadvantage of giving a white appearance to the skin on application may be overcome by incorporating these filters in microparticles and nanoparticles [8, 9].

Organic UV filters may cause skin irritation, allergic, and photoallergic contact dermatitis. They are lipophilic molecules that may be absorbed and accumulated in the adipose tissue, leading to systemic effects (endocrine-disrupting effects, cytotoxicity, neurotoxicity, and behavioral changes). Some compounds are unstable under exposure to ultraviolet radiation and may trigger phototoxic reactions, adding extra oxidative damage to skin cells [2, 10]. To mitigate this effect, different antioxidants (retinol, ascorbic acid, and tocopherol) have been included in sunscreen formulations [8]. Another disadvantage of conventional UV filters is the harmful effect on ecosystems, which negatively impacts the human body [4].

The demand for natural, safe, and sustainable alternatives to synthetic UV filters has driven significant interest in plant-based compounds and extracts for sunscreen formulations. These natural ingredients provide protection against ultraviolet (UV) radiation while often offering additional skin benefits, such as antioxidant and anti-inflammatory properties [2]. Some plant compounds contain chromophores that absorb UV radiation and convert it into harmless heat, similar to synthetic chemical filters. Plant compounds with aromatic rings usually show a broad absorption spectrum with a wavelength range of 200–400 nm [1].

Antioxidants present in plant extracts neutralize reactive oxygen species (ROS), mitigating the oxidative stress induced by UV radiation. Moreover, plant-derived compounds often possess anti-inflammatory properties that soothe the skin and reduce erythema (sunburn). Notable natural compounds that can be used in sunscreen formulations are polyphenols (epigallocatechin gallate from green tea; proanthocyanidins from grape seed; flavonoids like apigenin, quercetin, rutin, kaempferol; phenolic acids, such as ferulic acid and caffeic acid), carotenoids (beta-carotene, lycopene, and lutein), seed oils (shea butter, cocoa butter, jojoba oil, rosehip oil, and grapeseed oil), volatile oils (chamomile, lavender), and alkaloids (sanguinarine, piperine, and caffeine) [2, 11].

This chapter presents an overall profile of the plant extracts or compounds with UV-filter activity, their main biological effects, their mechanisms of anti-UV activity, and modern nano-formulations that can increase their activity. The review is based on articles published in the last 5 years, retrieved by searches of the following electronic databases: Web of Science, Pubmed, Google Scholar, Elsevier, and Wiley. Only articles including plant extracts or natural compounds from plant sources were selected. The following keywords were used: sunscreen, SPF, sun protection factor, and UV filter. All keywords were searched individually and in combination.

2. Plant-based UV protection agents in sunscreens

One of the primary benefits of plant extracts and compounds as UV filters is their natural ability to absorb and reflect harmful UV radiation. These phytochemicals work by either absorbing UV rays or acting as physical barriers to reduce the penetration of harmful radiation into the skin. Plant-based UV filters are often rich in antioxidants, which play a vital role in neutralizing free radicals caused by UV exposure, thereby helping to prevent skin aging and cellular damage [12]. These antioxidants can protect the skin from oxidative stress and inflammation, reducing the risk of sunburn, premature aging, and skin cancer. Unlike synthetic chemicals, plant extracts provide a more holistic form of protection by not only shielding the skin from UV damage but also supporting its recovery and regeneration [2].

One of the major concerns with conventional sunscreens is their use of potentially harmful synthetic chemicals, such as oxybenzone, avobenzone, and parabens. These chemicals can sometimes cause skin irritation, allergies, or hormonal disruptions [7]. In contrast, plant-based sunscreens are typically less likely to cause such adverse reactions. The natural origin of these compounds makes them more suitable for individuals with sensitive skin or those seeking to avoid exposure to harsh synthetic substances. For example, aloe gel is widely known for its soothing and anti-inflammatory properties, making it ideal for calming sunburned or irritated skin [13].

Another significant advantage of using plant extracts as sunscreens is their sustainability and minimal environmental impact. Many chemical-based sunscreens, particularly those containing oxybenzone and octinoxate, have been shown to harm marine life by contributing to coral reef degradation. Plant-based sunscreens, on the other hand, are biodegradable and typically have less harmful effects on the environment, making them a better option for eco-conscious consumers [14].

Plant name/natural compound	Type of extract and plant parts used	Mechanism of action	Formulations	Ref.
Agave americana var. americana (Aa) *A. americana var. marginata (Am)*	Ethanolic extract of leaves	Aa extract: SPF of 9.95; Am extract: SPF of 5.84; phytosome formulations with Aa extract had SPF activity of 9.96–13.3 (with 40 mg extract and 60 mg soy lecithin)	Formulations with phytosomes (with 20–40 mg dry ethanolic extract)	[15]
Aloe vera	*Aloe vera*-loaded solid liquid nanoparticles	*In vitro* SPF value of 16.9 ± 2.44; *in vivo* SPF value of 14.81 ± 3.81	Solid lipid nanoparticles	[16]
Astragalus monspessulanus	Ethanolic extract	SPF of 38.55 ± 0.85 due to antioxidant activity	—	[17]
Baccharis antioquensis	Polyphenol extracts from the leaves, in different solvents (ethanol, methanol, hexane, dichloromethane, ethyl acetate)	Highest SPF value (21.9 ± 3.3) was obtained for the methanolic extract	Oil-in-water (O/W) emulsions of the extracts alone or mixed	[18]
Buddleja salina (the false olive)	Ethanolic extract from leaves and stem	Antioxidant, antiproliferative activity against human dermal fibroblasts; SPF value of 16.1 and UVA protection factor (UVAPF) values of 6.45	O/W emulsion	[19]
Calceolarioside (CAL), myconoside (MYC), and *Haberlea rhodopensis* methanol extract (HRE)	Isolated from the leaves of *Haberlea rhodopensis*	HRE, MYC, and CAL significantly reduced intracellular ROS formation in UVR-exposed HaCaT cells; modulation of redox homeostasis; CAL is a potent natural NRF2 activator	—	[20]
Calea fruticosa	N-hexane, ethyl acetate, and ethanol aerial parts extracts	Highest SPF value (9.665) was obtained for the ethanolic extract (0.1 mg/mL) due to coumarin content and its antioxidant activity Extracts showed synergistic action on the sunscreen	Sunscreen UVA-UVB 5% Pemulen TR-1 gel mixed with the extracts	[21]
Carpobrotus edulis	Aqueous leaf extract	Photoprotective activity (absorption in UV region)	Oil in cream emulsion	[22]
Catechins	Isolated from *Uncaria gambir* leaves	Antioxidant properties SPF 16	O/W emulsion with *Cera alba*, tween 80, cetyl alcohol, and stearyl alcohol	[23]
Cistus ladanifer	Labdanum resin	Antiaging Anti-inflammatory activity due to its flavonoid fraction		[24]

Plant name/natural compound	Type of extract and plant parts used	Mechanism of action	Formulations	Ref.
Cocos nucifera	Ethanolic husk fiber extract	Photoprotection due to phenolic compounds	Emulsions of various concentrations of extract 5–20% in lanette base	[25]
Cocos nucifera	Dark and light-colored lignin from coconut husk	Light-colored lignin exhibits a higher level of UV absorption; Addition of 4% lignin into a commercial sunscreen led to nearly a twofold increase in SPF and UVAPF value	Combinations with plain cream and SPF cream (with various concentrations of lignin of both types)	[26]
Cyperus rotundus (nutsedge)	Aqueous extract of tubers	Antioxidant SPF 5.794	—	[27]
Calendula officinalis, Daucus carota, Solanum lycopersicum, Humulus lupulus	Marigold petals, carrot roots, tomato fruits, and hop cones (water/water and propylene glycol/oil extracts)	Antioxidant due to phenolic content; SPF determined by spectrophotometric method (hop water extract SPF 21)	—	[28]
Curcuma longa, Daucus carota, Camellia sinensis, Aloe vera, Cera flava, Cocos nucifera	Turmeric powder, carrot seeds, green tea extract, aloe gel, beeswax, coconut oil	Photoprotection due to compounds with antioxidant activity; SPF values of 33.43 and 33.50	Coconut oil-based sunscreens	[13]
Daucus carota	Carrot extract	Carrot extract was as effective as SPF 15 in preventing apoptosis of mouse fibroblasts exposed to UVB; an antioxidant	—	[29]
Daucus carota	Carrot seed oil	SPF value of 0.1 for the *in vitro* determination and 2.5 for the *in vivo* determination	—	[30]
Gamma-oryzanol, *Daucus carota, Vitellaria paradoxa, Cera flava*	Gamma-oryzanol-loaded NLCs, nanosized UV filters, carrot seed oil, shea butter, beeswax	SPF = 34 due to the presence of both inorganic and organic UV filters, the potent antioxidant gamma-oryzanol, and natural oils, with synergistic effects	Topical xanthan gum nanogel	[31]
Daucus carota	Carrot root extract, carrot seed oil, sunflower oil, canola oil, beta-carotene, tocopheryl aceatate	Photoprotection from blue light: in the 415—455 nm wavelength range associated with oxidative stress, Carotolino (0.4%) reduced blue light by 97%	Lipophilic complex (Carotolino)	[32]
Dalbergia sissoo	Leaves aqueous extract, fruits aqueous extract, bark aqueous extract	Leaves and fruit extracts have moderate SPF; bark extract has shown SPF value (39.38) higher than positive control (33.76); antioxidant, DNA protection, and anti-proliferative activity	Gel formulations with 1 mg/ml extract	[33]

Plant name/natural compound	Type of extract and plant parts used	Mechanism of action	Formulations	Ref.
Dihydroquercetin (DHQ) Quercetin (Q) Beta-carotene (βC)	—	Emulsion with 0.5% DHQ and 2% βC has SPF 5.19, emulsion with 0.5% DHQ has SPF 4.65, and emulsion with 0.5% Q has SPF 3.35	Fast inverted oil-in-water emulsion/ SWitch-Oil-Phase (SWOP) emulsions	[34]
Elaeagnus angustifolia	70% methanolic extract of leaves (EAPE)	SPF values of formulations with 2–8% EAPE was in the range of 6.37 ± 0.14 to 21.05 ± 0.85	Emulgel (emulsion type O/W) with EAPE, sesame oil, and sea buckthorn oil	[35]
Elaeocarpus floribundus	N-hexane, ethyl acetate, and methanol leaf extracts	Antioxidant activity; SPF values of methanol extract were 45.470, 44.791, 43.754, 38.861, and 21.102 for 1000, 800, 600, 400, and 200 μg /mL, respectively	—	[36]
Epigallocatechin gallate	Isolated from green tea leaves	Antioxidant activity protects fibroblasts from oxidative-stress damage; broad-spectrum UV absorption and lower UV transmittance than commercial sunscreens with SPF 15 and 30	Formulations with 10 wt% EA NPs (epigallocatechin gallate/ aminobenzoic acid nanoparticles)	[37]
Erica australis	Aqueous extract of flower	Antioxidant activity: Flower extracts showed a negligible SPF value (0.18). The elaborated sunscreen creams presented an SPF of 5.8	O/W emulsion	[38]
Helichrysum odoratissimum	The ethanolic extract of leaves and stem	Antioxidant, antiproliferative activity against human dermal fibroblasts; SPF value of 16.0 and UVAPF values of 6.47	O/W emulsion	[19]
Lignin obtained from *Kenaf* stalks (*Hibiscus cannabinus*)	Light-color lignin	2% lignin nanospheres added to SPF 30 sunscreen increased SPF value to 67.88; 4% lignin nanosphere added to SPF 10 sunscreen increased SPF to 27.84	Lignin nanospheres added to commercial sunscreen lotion of SPF 10 and 30	[39]
Moringa concanensis	Hexane, chloroform, methanol, and ethyl acetate stem bark extracts	Photoprotection due to antioxidant activity; SPF value of 10.50 ± 0.23 for the chloroform extract	—	[40]
Nephelium lappaceum (rambutan)	The ethanolic extract of fruit peel	Addition of rambutan total phenolics (at concentrations of 0.25%, 0.50%, and 1.00%) to organic sunscreens, resulting in an increase of SPF values of 23.5, 49.6, and 134.9%	Cream emulsions	[41]

Plant name/natural compound	Type of extract and plant parts used	Mechanism of action	Formulations	Ref.
Oncosiphon suffruticosum	Essential oil from the fresh aerial parts	SPF value of 2.299 photoprotection due to antioxidant activity	—	[42]
Opuntia ficus-indica (prickly pear)	Seed pomace extracts (a by-product of seed oil extraction)	SPF value of 8.36 ± 0.53; photoprotection due to antioxidant activity	Oil-in-water emulsions	[43]
Orbignya phalerata (babassu)	Lipophilic extract of seeds	SPF of 35.5 ± 3.0, photostable after 6 h of radiation and non-cytotoxic to fibroblast cells	Oil-in-water nanoemulsion containing babassu lipophilic extract and low concentrations of organic sunscreens	[44]
P-coumaric acid	—	SPF value of 36 ± 0.2 and UVAPF value of 16 ± 0.4; significant reduction of UV-A induced oxidative stress biomarkers; enhanced permeation	*P*-coumaric acid-phospholipid complex-loaded gel	[45]
Pluchea discoridis, Lawsonia inermis, Aloe vera, Eucalyptus camaldulensis	90% methanolic extract of leaves	Antioxidant activity: Extracts (1 mg/ml) had SPF values of 18.79 ± 2.01, 19.97 ± 0.78, 18.85 ± 1.10, and 17.97 ± 1.24, respectively	—	[46]
Psidium guajava	Ethanolic fruit extract	Photoprotection due to the flavonoid and tannin content improved the photoprotection of an organic filter formulation with 134% (SPF 8.1)	Cream with guava-fruit extract and 2-ethyl-hexyl methoxycinnamate	[47]
Punica granatum	Polyphenol enriched fraction (PEF) of pomegranate peel	Antioxidant activity; SPF value of 7.5; UV-A1/total UV value of 0.94	Water-in-oil emulsions with 5% zinc oxide-PEF nanoparticles	[48]
Punica granatum	Pomegranate seed oil	Cell DNA protection against UVB-induced damage	Pomegranate seed oil nanoemulsion with pomegranate peel polyphenol-rich extract encapsulation	[11]
Rutin	—	Reduced skin erythema, increased UVA radiation photoprotection	Gelatin nanostructures	[49]
Salsola foetida	Methanolic extract of dried aerial parts	SPF values of 21.3 ± 0.03 due to high content of phenols, flavonoids (anthocyanins), and antioxidant and anti-inflammatory effect	—	[50]
Schinus terebinthifolius	Ethanolic fruit peel extract (STPE) and ethanolic whole fruit extract (STWFE)	SPF values of 20.15–26.82 for STPE and 5.08–16.41 for STWFE; SPF values of emulsion extracts varied between 1.25 and 32.40 for STPE and 0.52 and 41.58 for STWFE	Emulsion of STPE or STWFE of 5% or 10% concentration in Lanette base	[51]

Plant name/natural compound	Type of extract and plant parts used	Mechanism of action	Formulations	Ref.
Spondias purpurea	70% v/v ethanolic extract of stem bark	SPF value for the extract (14.37 at 0.2 mg/mL and 26.16 at 2 mg/mL); SPF values of the formulations obtained in 0.2 mg mL^{-1} (0.495–2.27) and 2.0 mg mL^{-1} (2.29–15.87); antioxidant activity due to phenolic content	Formulations with different concentrations (0.2–10% ethanolic extract of stem bark)	[52]
Stenochlaena palustris (kelakai)	70% ethanolic extract of root	SPF value of 9.816; erythema transmission percentage of 9.591%; pigmentation transmission percentage of 16.779%	0.5% microemulsion (with 0.1% extract) incorporated into a gel form	[53]

Table 1.
Plants and natural compounds with photoprotective activity.

Some plant compounds, such as the polyphenols found in red algae and certain fruits, provide broad-spectrum protection against both UVA and UVB rays. By using plant-based sunscreens, consumers benefit from natural compounds that can offer protection across the full spectrum of UV radiation. Their antioxidant properties, non-toxic nature, and broad-spectrum protection make them a valuable option for consumers looking to protect their skin from harmful UV rays while also promoting overall skin health [1]. **Table 1** lists plants and phytocompounds that have been investigated as active sunscreen ingredients in the last 5 years.

Despite their advantages, natural compounds used in sunscreens face certain challenges: lower SPF, stability issues, variability in efficacy, skin penetration, cost and scalability, and regulatory approval. Most natural extracts provide moderate sun protection factors, often insufficient for high-performance sunscreens. As a result, they are typically combined with synthetic filters to meet regulatory standards for sun protection [54].

Many natural compounds degrade rapidly under prolonged UV exposure, reducing their effectiveness over time. Stabilizing these ingredients often requires advanced formulation techniques or the addition of synthetic stabilizers, which may reduce their appeal as “natural” products [54].

The photoprotective efficacy of plant-based ingredients can vary significantly depending on factors such as plant species, extraction method, and formulation. This variability poses challenges for standardization and consistent performance. In addition, some natural UV filters struggle to penetrate the skin adequately to provide effective protection, limiting their functionality in topical applications. **Also,** the extraction and purification of high-quality natural compounds can be expensive and resource-intensive, making it difficult to scale production for commercial use [55].

Regulatory frameworks for sunscreen products often require rigorous testing of efficacy and safety. There are no natural compounds approved as UV filters in the European Union or USA [14]. Many natural extracts lack the extensive scientific validation needed to obtain approval, delaying their adoption in mainstream sunscreen products.

3. Enhanced sunscreen formulations

Plant extracts and isolated plant compounds have been included over time in various classic formulations (emulsions, microemulsions, conventional gels, creams) or modern ones with the aim of increasing their stability, their ability to spread and penetrate the skin, and improving their organoleptic appearance, but also to make them as easy to apply as possible and as attractive as possible for those who use them.

The development of new eco-friendly formulations from renewable sources represents an increased concern in obtaining cosmeceuticals. Classical sunscreen formulations predominantly consist of popular emulsion-based products, such as creams, gel creams, and lotions. Water-in-oil (w/o) emulsions are often favored for sunscreens due to their ability to deliver high SPF and excellent water resistance. However, w/o emulsions typically contain a higher oil-to-water ratio, resulting in a greasy texture and heavier feel, which can make them less appealing compared to oil-in-water (o/w) emulsions. To address this, fast-inverting o/w emulsions, also known as Switch-Oil-Phase (SWOP) emulsions, have been developed. These emulsions invert into w/o emulsions upon application, forming a lipophilic, water-resistant layer on the skin, making them particularly suitable for sun protection products. Thus, Radava Martić et al. tested the antioxidant activity and UV absorption of several SWOP emulsions added with dihydroquercetin and ß-carotene [34]. The SPF of SWOP emulsion that consisted of combining dihydroquercetin and ß-carotene was the highest (5.19), likely due to the combined effect of both active ingredients. While β-carotene is not a conventional UV absorber, it may protect dihydroquercetin from oxidation through its antioxidant properties, thereby enhancing dihydroquercetin's UV absorbance. In contrast, the SPF of the emulsion base S was minimal. These results highlight the good photoprotective potential of the selected antioxidants when combined with a promising cosmetic carrier like the SWOP emulsion [34].

Isolated constituents from the crude plant extracts have demonstrated greater photoprotection capacity compared to the extract. It is the case of two phenylethanoid glycosides (calceolarioside and myconoside), isolated from *Haberlea rhodopensis* leaves. These compounds could be used in photoprotective formulations, given their ability to reduce UVA/UVB-induced ROS production, results observed in an in vitro photoaging model in human keratinocytes. It appears that calceolarioside is a potent NRF2 activator; meanwhile, myconoside stimulates PGC-1α and TGF-1β/SMAD/Wnt signaling pathways [20].

The association of coconut oil with *Aloe vera* gel, turmeric, green tea, and carrot seed led to a more improved formula, with a protection factor of 33.47. The topical preparation presented a good safety profile for topical application without mutagenic effects, irritation, or erythema. In addition, it proved to be homogeneous, uniform, stable, and presented *in vitro* a good antioxidant activity [13].

But there are also cases where the addition of a plant extract to a commercial UV filter with a known protection factor does not result in an improvement in SPF, possibly due to the lack of synergism between the components. Rodrigues et al. managed to identify a large number of compounds in the stem bark extract of *Spondias purpurea* (phenolic acids, tannins, flavonoids and derivatives, and benzophenones), which explained the high antioxidant activity. Also, the SPF value of the extract was higher (26.16) than that of octyl methoxycinnamate (SPF 21.84), a substance known for its photoprotective effect. Unexpectedly, in the formulation that combined the two, a decrease in SPF by 9 units (17.16) was detected. However, plant extracts are valuable sources of compounds that can prevent cellular degradation following exposure to UV radiation, thus contributing to greater skin protection [52].

3.1 Oil-in-water emulsions

Oil-in-water emulsions (O/W) are frequently used in cosmeceuticals and have high potential for several industrial areas (pharmaceuticals, cosmetics, and food). In the cosmetics industry, water-in-oil emulsions are used in creams and lotions, provding a hydrating effect and helping deliver moisture deep into the skin. These emulsions are particularly effective in creating products that offer long-lasting moisture without feeling greasy, and plant extracts can be easily included in such formulations [56].

An emulgel containing different concentrations of *Elaeagnus angustifolia* purified extract from leaves (2, 4, 6, 8%) proved to have good stability for 8 weeks in temperature variations between 4 and 40°C. The preliminary tests regarding stability led to the conclusion that the best concentration was 6%, and this formulation had colorless effects on the skin. The sun protective factor (SPF) for this new emulsion O/W was spectrophotometrically detected, and its value of 16.03 makes this species a good, natural candidate as an alternative to synthetic substances, thus reducing adverse reactions [35]. According to the European Cosmetic Regulation 1223/2009, the protection categories based on the SPF results (*in vitro* or *in vivo* tests) are the following: measured SPF 6–14.9 (low protection), SPF 15–29.9 (medium protection), and SPF 30–59.9 (high protection) [57].

Buddleja salina and *Helichrysum odoratissimum* are another two plants with antioxidant activity and antiproliferative effects against skin cancer lines. The ethanolic extracts of leaves and stems of these species were incorporated in two O/W emulsions, to which was also added titanium dioxide (Solaveil™ XT-100), in order to obtain an SPF of 15. The ethanolic plant extracts were added in an amount of 6.0 mg/mL in each formulation and represented 10% of the ingredients. The good results obtained in the *in vivo* skin irritation tests on female volunteers (18–65 years old), but also the test on the human dermal fibroblast cell line, which attests to non-mutagenicity, correlated with an SPF of approximately 16 and UVAPF (UVA protection factor) of 6.45 for *B. salina* and 6.47 for *H. odoratissimum*, making the two plants valuable sources of natural ingredients added to products with a photoprotective effect [19].

3.2 Microemulsions

Microemulsions are also used in the cosmetics industry to improve skin penetration. They are thermodynamically stable mixtures of oil, water, and surfactants, characterized by their nanoscale droplet size [58].

The 70% ethanolic extract of roots of *Stenochlaena palustris* with a high content of flavonoids, alkaloids, and saponins have proven their efficiency in terms of UV protection of the skin when incorporated into a microemulsion gel. In addition, the gel formulated with sodium carboxymethyl cellulose and propylene glycol was classified as "sunblock" in the tests regarding evaluation of erythema transmission percentage and pigmentation transmission percentage [53].

3.3 Nanostructures

The increasing awareness of the need for effective sun protection has driven innovation in sunscreen formulations, with nanostructures emerging as a game-changing technology. Nanostructured systems, such as nanoparticles, liposomes, and nanoemulsions, have transformed sunscreen development, particularly with plant-based compounds and extracts as active ingredients. These advanced formulations offer enhanced UV protection, stability, and environmental sustainability [59]. Nanostructures protect delicate plant compounds, like polyphenols and flavonoids, from degradation by light, oxygen, or heat, ensuring prolonged efficacy [4]. Liposomes and solid lipid nanoparticles transport active compounds like curcumin or resveratrol deeper into the skin, providing sustained protection and reducing the need for frequent reapplication [10]. Phytochemicals serve as safer, biodegradable alternatives to synthetic UV filters, minimizing environmental and health risks. Nanostructured formulations create lightweight, transparent, and non-greasy sunscreens, masking odors and textures of plant extracts for a better user experience [8]. These systems combine UV protection with skin benefits like hydration, antiaging, and anti-inflammatory effects, addressing diverse consumer needs. Efficient use of natural resources and biodegradable ingredients reduces the ecological footprint of sunscreens, especially in marine environments [60].

Advanced research in the field of dermatocosmetics has led to the development of formulations with phytosomes to improve the absorption of molecules into the skin. One such study conducted on ethanolic extract from *Agave americana* leaves showed that with increasing concentration of plant extract in phytosomes, an increase in SPF was also observed. In order to obtain phytosomes, varying concentrations of soy lecithin (50–70 mg), plant extract (20–40 mg), and 10 mg cholesterol, all dissolved in dichloromethane, were used. The formulated samples exhibited *in vitro* SPF values, ranging from 3.86 (control) to 9.96 (formulation with 20 mg extract), 12.2 (formulation with 30 mg extract), and 13.3 (formulation with 40 mg extract) [15].

Also, oil-in-water nanoemulsions prepared by ultrasound have been developed with the aim of increasing the solubility and stability of lipophilic substances or extracts. One such example is *Orbignya phalerata* lipophilic extract from seeds with a high content of saturated fatty acids (lauric acid 52.64% and myristic acid 15.42%), phenolic compounds, and tocopherols, which was incorporated into an oil-in-water nanoemulsion along with 4 substances known for their photoprotective effect. The authors of the study observed an increase in SPF from 28.6 (in the case of the preparation with benzophenone-3, diethylamino hydroxybenzoyl hexyl benzoate, octocrylene, and octyl methoxycinnamate) to 35.5 when babassu lipophilic extract was added. Although the formulation that included only the plant extract presented SPF < 2, it seems that the synergism of action between the components led to a more efficient photoprotective preparation, due to the plant compounds with antioxidant effect [44].

Reis-Mansur et al. proposed preparing some oil-in-water nanoemulsions with 3% buriti oil (*Mauritia flexuosa*) and 10% concentrated dry extract of *Aloe vera* spray-dried. The formulation named NE-A19, to which they added two synthetic filters (octyl methoxycinnamate and ethylhexyl methoxycrylene), proved to have satisfactory organoleptic properties, good stability, no phase separation and was safe for administration. Moreover, the SPF value was 49 [61].

Yingren Liu et al. produced lignin nanospheres for further use in cosmetic sunscreen formulations. The extracted stabilized lignin was dissolved in a gamma-valerolactone solution to achieve a concentration of 0.4 mg/mL. The resulting lignin solution was transferred into a dialysis bag and dialyzed at room temperature for 48 hours. Following this, the extracted lignin was vacuum-dried, and the lignin nanospheres were obtained. The morphology and particle size of the lignin nanospheres were measured by scanning electron microscope and a zeta potential tester. Lignin usually has a darker color, but the one obtained by this group of researchers has a lighter color, making it easier to use in cosmetic formulations [39].

P-coumaric acid is a hydroxycinnamic acid widely distributed in plants (fruits, beans, potatoes, tea) that has antioxidant and anti-inflammatory activity, inhibiting UV-B radiation and melanogenesis in cell line culture, but also having a UV-A protective effect. Unfortunately, it lacks the capacity to penetrate the deeper layers of the skin for a longer period of time. In this perspective, Biswas et al. have formulated a complexation of a p-coumaric acid with phospholipid hydrogenated soybean phosphatidylcholine in order to increase its permeability to the skin and its stability. This complex was incorporated in a gel base (carbopol 940) and tested by spectrophotometric methods to determine its SPF value, UV-A protection factor, and photo-stability. The gel met all the conditions for topical application, and the incorporation of coumaric acid in a complex increased the penetration capacity into the skin by almost 6 times. In addition, this formulation has a high capacity to protect the skin from UV radiation: SPF 35.5 and UVAPF 16.2 [45].

Rutin, a therapeutically active flavonoid, has been shown to possess a wide range of pharmacological activities, including anti-inflammatory, antimicrobial, and anticancer. However, its poor aqueous solubility, low membrane permeability, and bioavailability limit its therapeutic applications. In order to increase the penetration of the ingredient into deeper layers of the skin and its benefits in photoprotective formulations, rutin was frequently associated with nanostructures (ethosome, gelatin nanocapsules, phytosome, nanocrystal, chitosan/tripolyphosphate nanoparticles). The encapsulation of rutin into gelatin nanostructures and association with three known UV filters (ethylhexyl dimethyl PABA, ethylhexyl methoxycinnamate, and butyl methoxydibenzoylmethane) increased the *in vitro* value of SPF due to a possible synergistic effect among constituents [49].

Gamma-oryzanol (GO) is a plant-derived natural antioxidant composed of a mixture of more than ten phytosterol ferulates. Its antioxidant activity is considered to be up to 10 times stronger than that of vitamin E in rice bran. Beyond its potent antioxidant properties, gamma-oryzanol offers potential skin-protective benefits, including UV light absorption, intrinsic sun protection factor (SPF)-boosting capabilities, and reported antiaging effects. Badalkhani et al. developed a topical nanogel containing gamma-oryzanol-loaded nanostructured lipid carriers (NLCs) and nanosized UV filters (TiO_2 and methylene bis-benzotriazolyl tetramethylbutylphenol). This involved partially replacing UV filters by incorporating and maximizing the amount of the powerful plant-derived antioxidant (gamma-oryzanol) in the formulations. The findings indicate that encapsulating GO into the NLCs did not result in an increase in particle size, instability, or a reduction in the uniformity of the nanoparticles. Thus, the formulation retained its desirable properties. The optimized nanosystem showed long-term stability and high photoprotection capacity (SPF = 34), along with no sensitization or skin irritation [31].

Aloe vera-loaded solid lipid nanoparticles formulated by Rodrigues et al. using glyceryl monostearate (300 mg) as a lipid and 100 mg aloe powder did not cause skin irritation or sensitization reactions in *in vivo* tests performed on Wistar albino rats. In addition, both *in vitro* and *in vivo* SPF tests showed good skin protection against UV light exposure (SPF = 16.9, respectively 14.81) [16].

The association of a plant such as *aloe vera* which has demonstrated photoprotection, with other plant extracts can lead to the development and innovation of much improved formulations. This is also the case of *Crocus sativus* (safranal)-loaded solid lipid nanoparticles (SLN), which were incorporated into a cream with aloe vera gel and almond oil. This product demonstrated good stability and excellent rheological properties, having an SPF of 9.22 [62].

4. Conclusions

Natural compounds and plant extracts offer promising alternatives to synthetic UV filters, combining photoprotection with additional skin benefits. Ingredients such as polyphenols, flavonoids, carotenoids, and oils have demonstrated efficacy in absorbing UV radiation, neutralizing oxidative stress, and reducing inflammation. However, challenges such as lower SPF values and stability issues must be addressed to optimize their use in commercial sunscreens. Continued research and innovation are essential to harness the full potential of these natural solutions.

The development of modern instrumental analysis methods and those assessing the biological activity of plant extracts and natural compounds has led to the creation of eco-friendly formulations in the cosmetics industry, offering multiple benefits for users. Innovations in dermatocosmetic formulations represent a significant step forward, especially as they have demonstrated the absence of adverse reactions, good skin tolerability, and additional effects in protecting the skin barrier against the harmful effects of UV radiation due to their antioxidant and anti-inflammatory properties. The development of sunscreen products based on plant extracts, either alone or in combination with synthetic substances known as UV filters, is continuously growing. Progress in this field supports consumers by offering sustainable products derived either from raw materials that are by-products of the wood industry or from renewable sources.

Nanostructured formulations represent a significant advancement in sunscreen technology, particularly when harnessing the power of plant-based compounds and extracts. By improving stability, enhancing delivery, reducing chemical load, and providing multifunctional benefits, these systems offer a superior alternative to traditional formulations. As consumer preference shifts toward safer, more sustainable products, nanostructured sunscreens incorporating natural compounds are poised to become the future of sun protection.

Conflict of interest

The authors declare no conflict of interest.

Author details

Cristina Lungu*, Adina Catinca Grădinaru and Bianca Ivănescu
Faculty of Pharmacy, "Grigore T. Popa," Department of Pharmaceutical Botany, University of Medicine and Pharmacy, Iasi, Romania

*Address all correspondence to: ape3_c@yahoo.com

References

[1] Li L, Chong L, Huang T, Ma Y, et al. Natural products and extracts from plants as natural UV filters for sunscreens: A review. Animal Models and Experimental Medicine. 2023;**6**(3):183-195. DOI: 10.1002/ame2.12295

[2] Verma A, Zanoletti A, Kareem KY, Adelodun B, et al. Skin protection from solar ultraviolet radiation using natural compounds: A review. Environmental Chemistry Letters. 2024;**22**:273-295. DOI: 10.1007/s10311-023-01649-4

[3] Abou-Dahech M, Boddu SHS, Bachu RD, Babu RJ, et al. A mini-review on limitations associated with UV filters. Arabian Journal of Chemistry. 2022;**15**(11):104212. DOI: 10.1016/j.arabjc.2022.104212

[4] Fonseca M, Rehman M, Soares R, Fonte P. The impact of flavonoid-loaded nanoparticles in the UV protection and safety profile of topical sunscreens. Biomolecules. 2023;**13**(3):493. DOI: 10.3390/biom13030493

[5] Gracia-Cazaña T, Aguilera J, Navarro-Bielsa A, González S, Lim HW, Gilaberte Y. New trends on personalized sunscreens. Photodermatology, Photoimmunology & Photomedicine. 2024;**40**(3):e12967. DOI: 10.1111/phpp.12967

[6] Ferreira L, Torres B, Hameed H, Vieira ACF, et al. Updated insights of active cosmetic ingredients against blue light: *In vivo* and *in vitro* evidence. Journal of Drug Delivery Science and Technology. 2024;**101**(B):106306. DOI: 10.1016/j.jddst.2024.106306

[7] Huang Y, Law J, Lam T, Leung K. Risks of organic UV filters: A review of environmental and human health concern studies. Science of the Total Environment. 2021;**755**(1):142486. DOI: 10.1016/j.scitotenv.2020.142486

[8] Santos A, Marto J, Chá-Chá R, Martins AM, et al. Nanotechnology-based sunscreens - a review. Materials Today Chemistry. 2022;**23**:100709. DOI: 10.1016/j.mtchem.2021.100709

[9] Mascarenhas-Melo F, Mathur A, Murugappan S, Sharma A, et al. Inorganic nanoparticles in dermopharmaceutical and cosmetic products: Properties, formulation development, toxicity, and regulatory issues. European Journal of Pharmaceutics and Biopharmaceutics. 2023;**192**:25-40. DOI: 10.1016/j.ejpb.2023.09.011

[10] Júnior JADC, Mendonça Santos A, Santos Oliveira AM, Santos AB, et al. Use of nanotechnology applied to sunscreens: Technological prospection based on patents. Journal of Drug Delivery Science and Technology. 2024;**91**:105245. DOI: 10.1016/j.jddst.2023.105245

[11] Chu CC, Nyam KL. Application of seed oils and its bioactive compounds in sunscreen formulations. Journal of the American Oil Chemists' Society. 2021;**98**:713-726. DOI: 10.1002/aocs.12491

[12] Mansuri R, Diwan A, Kumar H, Dangwal K, Yadav D. Potential of natural compounds as sunscreen agents. Pharmacognosy Reviews. 2021;**15**(29):47-56. DOI: 10.5530/phrev.2021.15.5

[13] Tiwari R, Singh I, Gupta M, Singh LP, et al. Formulation and evaluation of herbal sunscreens: An assessment towards skin protection from ultraviolet radiation. Pharmacophore.

2023;**13**(3):41-49. DOI: 10.51847/svzLRFMP5F

[14] Milutinov J, Pavlović N, Ćirin D, Atanacković Krstonošić M, Krstonošić V. The potential of natural compounds in UV protection products. Molecules. 2024;**29**(22):5409. DOI: 10.3390/molecules29225409

[15] Vaghela H, Mbatia B, Calvin A, Sania F, et al. Formulation of phytosomes with sun protection factor using *Agave americana* ethanolic extract. Journal of Biologically Active Products from Nature. 2024;**14**:238-250. DOI: 10.1080/22311866.2024.2335153

[16] Rodrigues LR, Jose J. Exploring the photo protective potential of solid lipid nanoparticle-based sunscreen cream containing *Aloe vera*. Environmental Science and Pollution Research International. 2020;**27**(17):20876-20888. DOI: 10.1007/s11356-020-08543-4

[17] Benslama O, Lekmine S, Mansouri N. Phytochemical constituents of *Astragalus monspessulanus* and integrative analysis for its antioxidant, photoprotective, and antityrosinase activities: Experimental and computational investigation. European Journal of Integrative Medicine. 2023;**60**:102247. DOI: 10.1016/j.eujim.2023.102247

[18] Monsalve-Bustamante YA, López Figueroa F, Vega J, Rodrigues Moreira B, et al. Holistic photoprotection, broad spectrum (UVA-UVB), and biological effective protection factors (BEPFs) from *Baccharis antioquensis* hydrolysates polyphenols. Plants. 2023;**12**(5):979. DOI: 10.3390/plants12050979

[19] Twilley D, Moodley D, Rolfes H, Moodley I, McGawd L, et al. Ethanolic extracts of south African plants, *Buddleja saligna* wild. and *Helichrysum odoratissimum* (L.) sweet, as multifunctional ingredients in sunscreen formulations. South African Journal of Botany. 2021;**137**:171-182. DOI: 10.1016/j.sajb.2020.10.010

[20] Stoykova ID, Koycheva IK, Binev BK, Mihaylova LV, et al. Myconoside and calceolarioside E restrain UV-induced skin photoaging by activating NRF2-mediated defense mechanisms. International Journal of Molecular Sciences. 2024;**25**:2441. DOI: 10.3390/ijms25042441

[21] Seregheti TMQ, Pinto APR, da Goncalves CM, dos Antunes SA, et al. Antiproliferative and photoprotective activities of the extracts and compounds from *Calea fruticosa*. Brazilian Journal of Medical and Biological Research. 2020;**53**(9):e9375. DOI: 10.1590/1414-431X20209375

[22] Lassoued MA, Ben Fatma NH, Romdhane MH, Faidi A, et al. Photoprotective potential of a Tunisian halophyte plant *Carpobrotus edulis* L. European Journal of Integrative Medicine. 2021;**42**(1):101286. DOI: 10.1016/j.eujim.2021.101286

[23] Mita SR, Husni P, Putriana NA, Maharani R, et al. A recent update on the potential use of catechins in cosmeceuticals. Cosmetics. 2024;**11**:23. DOI: 10.3390/cosmetics11010023

[24] Frazão DF, Martins-Gomes C, Steck JL, Keller J, et al. Labdanum resin from *Cistus ladanifer* L.: A natural and sustainable ingredient for skin care cosmetics with relevant cosmeceutical bioactivities. Plants (Basel). 2022;**11**:1477. DOI: 10.3390/plants11111477

[25] Oliveira MBS, Valentim IB, Santos TR, Xavier JA, et al. Photoprotective and antiglycation activities of non-toxic *Cocos nucifera* Linn. (Arecaceae) husk fiber ethanol

extract and its phenol chemical composition. Industrial Crops and Products. 2021;**162**:113246. DOI: 10.1016/j.indcrop.2021.113246

[26] van Duy N, Tsygankov PY, Menshutina NV. Facile lignin extraction and application as natural UV blockers in cosmetic formulations. Chemical Engineering. 2024;**8**:69. DOI: 10.3390/chemengineering8040069

[27] Ben Ali A, Chouikh A, Haddad L. *Cyperus rotundus* tubers resin from Algeria: A promising source of natural antioxidants, anti-inflammatory, and photoprotective compounds. Ovidius University Annals of Chemistry. 2023;**34**:132-139. DOI: 10.2478/auoc-2023-0017

[28] Kurzawa M, Wilczynska E, Brudzynska P, Sionkowska A. Total phenolic content, antioxidant capacity and UV radiation protection properties of marigold (*Calendula officinalis*), carrot (*Daucus carota*), tomato (*Solanum lycopersicum*) and hop (*Humulus lupulus*) extracts. Cosmetics. 2022;**9**:134. DOI: 10.3390/cosmetics9060134

[29] Satriyasa BK, Widianti IGA, Fajar Manuaba IBG. The potential of carrot extract as a sunscreen to prevent apoptosis in white mice (*Mus musculus*) fibroblast cell cultures exposed to UVB light. Bali Medical Journal. 2022;**11**(2):527-530. DOI: 10.15562/bmj.v11i2.3460

[30] Ácsová A, Hojerová J, Janotková L, Bendová H, et al. The real UVB photoprotective efficacy of vegetable oils: *In vitro* and *in vivo* studies. Photochemical & Photobiological Sciences. 2021;**20**:139-151. DOI: 10.1007/s43630-020-00009-3

[31] Badalkhani O, Pires PC, Mohammadi M, Babaie S, et al. Nanogel containing gamma-oryzanol-loaded nanostructured lipid carriers and TiO_2/MBBT: A synergistic nanotechnological approach of potent natural antioxidants and nanosized UV filters for skin protection. Pharmaceuticals. 2023;**16**:670. DOI: 10.3390/ph16050670

[32] Martiniaková S, Hojerová J, Turányiová Z, Dvoranová D, et al. Reducing the impact of artificial blue light on the skin: A spectroscopic study. Acta Chimica Slovenica. 2024;**17**(1):55-62. DOI: 10.2478/acs-2024-0007

[33] Shagufta Y, Promila G. Cosmeceutical and anticancer potential of aqueous extracts of *Dalbergia sissoo* Roxb. aerial parts. Journal of Herbal Medicine. 2021;**29**:100456. DOI: 10.1016/j.hermed.2021.100456

[34] Martić R, Kotur-Stevuljević J, Malenović A, Ušjak L, et al. Fast inverted photoprotective o/w emulsionsloaded with dihydroquercetin and β-carotene: An innovative approach to *in vitro* assessment of antioxidant activity in a bioenvironment. Natural Product Communications. 2022;**17**:1-12. DOI: 10.1177/1934578X221112811

[35] Ahmady A, Amini MH, Zhakfar AM, Babak G, Sediqi MN. Sun protective potential and physical stability of herbal sunscreen developed from Afghan medicinal plants. Turkish Journal of Pharmaceutical Sciences. 2020;**17**:285-292. DOI: 10.4274/tjps.galenos.2019.15428

[36] Utami R, Syahputra R, Dona R, Fadhli H, et al. Total flavonoid content and *in vitro* study on the sunscreen activity of extracts of leaves of *Elaeocarpus floribundus* blume. Pharmacy Education. 2023;**23**:118-121. DOI: 10.46542/pe.2023.232.118121

[37] Chen X, Yi Z, Chen G, Ma X, Tong Q, Tang L, et al. Engineered fabrication

of EGCG-UV absorber conjugated nano-assemblies for antioxidative sunscreens with broad-band absorption. Colloids and Surfaces. B, Biointerfaces. 2022;**220**:112912. DOI: 10.1016/j.colsurfb.2022.112912

[38] López-Hortas L, Conde E, Falqué E, Domínguez H, Torres MD. Antioxidant capacity of the extracts from flowers of *Erica australis* L.: Comparison between microwave hydro diffusion and gravity (MHG) and distillation extraction techniques - formulation of sunscreen creams. Industrial Crops and Products. 2020;**145**:112079. DOI: 10.1016/j.indcrop.2019.112079

[39] Yingren L, Xing-Xiang J, Zhongjian T, Hairui J, et al. A cascade valorization of Kenaf stalk for the preparation of lignin sunscreens and papermaking. International Journal of Biological Macromolecules. 2023;**230**:123122. DOI: 10.1016/j.ijbiomac.2022.123122

[40] Santhanam R, Karunakaran T, Sowndhararajan K, Zulkifli MF, et al. Photoprotective potential, cytotoxicity, and UPLC-QTOF/MS analysis on bioactive solvent fractions of *Moringa concanensis* Nimmo bark. eCAM. 2022;**2022**:3781189. DOI: 10.1155/2022/3781189

[41] Mota MD, da Boa Morte AN, Silva LCRCE, Chinalia FA. Sunscreen protection factor enhancement through supplementation with Rambutan (*Nephelium lappaceum* L) ethanolic extract. Journal of Photochemistry and Photobiology. B. 2020;**205**:111837. DOI: 10.1016/j.jphotobiol.2020.111837

[42] Adewinogo SO, Sharma R, Africa CJ, Marnewick JL, et al. Chemical composition and cosmeceutical potential of the essential oil of *Oncosiphon suffruticosum* (L.) Källersjö. Plants. 2021;**10**:1315. DOI: 10.3390/plants10071315

[43] Ferreira RM, Flórez-Fernández N, Silva AS, Saraiva JA, et al. *Opuntia ficus-indica* seed pomace extracts with high UV-screening ability in a circular economy approach for body lotions with solar protection. Journal of Industrial and Engineering Chemistry. 2024;**130**:456-467. DOI: 10.1016/j.jiec.2023.09.052

[44] Vieira IRS, Lima Nunes Silva A, Castro N, Pinto C, et al. Development and characterization of photoprotective nanoemulsions containing Babassu (*Orbignya phalerata* Mart.) lipophilic extract. Brazilian Journal of Pharmaceutical Sciences. 2023;**59**:e23011. DOI: 10.1590/s2175-97902023e23011

[45] Biswas S, Mukherjee PK, Kar A, Bannerjee S, et al. Enhanced permeability and photoprotective potential of optimized p-coumaric acid-phospholipid complex loaded gel against UVA mediated oxidative stress. Journal of Photochemistry and Photobiology. B. 2021;**221**:112246. DOI: 10.1016/j.jphotobiol.2021.112246

[46] Mohamed A, Sorour W. Assessment of photoprotective, antioxidant and anti-skin cancer activities of leaf extracts of certain medicinal plants. Egyptian Journal of Botany. 2020;**60**:749-762. DOI: 10.21608/ejbo.2020.26982.1480

[47] Mota MD, Costa RYS, Guedes AAS, Silva LCRCE, Chinalia FA. Guava-fruit extract can improve the UV-protection efficiency of synthetic filters in sun cream formulations. Journal of Photochemistry and Photobiology. B. 2019;**201**:111639. DOI: 10.1016/j.jphotobiol.2019.111639

[48] Kokabi M, Ebrahimi SN. Polyphenol enriched extract of pomegranate peel; a

novel precursor for the nbiosynthesis of zinc oxide nanoparticles and application in sunscreens. Pharmaceutical Sciences. 2021;**27**(1):102-110. DOI: 10.34172/PS.2020.56

[49] Ariede MB, Gomez Junior WA, Cândido TM, de Aguiar MMGB, et al. Would rutin be a feasible strategy for environmental-friendly photoprotective samples? A review from stability to skin permeability and efficacy in sunscreen systems. Cosmetics. 2024;**11**:141. DOI: 10.3390/cosmetics11040141

[50] Gheraissa N, Elkhalifa Chemsa A, Cherrada N, Benamor B, et al. Exploring the phytochemical and biological properties of *Salsola foetida*: A promising wild plant from southeastern Algeria. International Journal of Food Properties. 2024;**27**(1):584-601. DOI: 10.1080/10942912.2024.2339248

[51] Oliveira MBS, Valentim IB, Rocha TS, Santosc JC, et al. *Schinus terebenthifolius* Raddi extracts: From sunscreen activity toward protection of the placenta to Zika virus infection, new uses for a well-known medicinal plant. Industrial Crops and Products. 2020;**152**:112503. DOI: 10.1016/j.indcrop.2020.112503

[52] Rodrigues F, Giffony P, Santos S, Guedes J, et al. *Spondias purpurea* L. stem bark extract: Antioxidant and *in vitro* photoprotective activities. Journal of the Brazilian Chemical Society. 2021;**32**:1918-1930. DOI: 21577/0103-5053.20210082

[53] ForestryanaD,RamadhanH,MaulidaP. The photoprotective effectiveness of microemulsion gel made from an ethanol extract of kelakai root (*Stenochlaena palustris* (Brum. f) Bedd.). Pharmacy Education. 2024;**24**:134-143. DOI: 10.46542/pe.2024.246.134143

[54] He H, Li A, Li S, Tang J, Li L, Xiong L. Natural components in sunscreens: Topical formulations with sun protection factor (SPF). Biomedicine & Pharmacotherapy. 2021;**134**:111161. DOI: 10.1016/j.biopha.2020.111161

[55] Shah Y, Mewada R. Recent advances in sunscreen agents and their formulations: A review. International Journal of Pharmaceutical Chemistry and Analysis. 2022;**9**(4):141-150. DOI: 10.18231/j.ijpca.2022.027

[56] Fresneda M, Trujillo-Cayado L, García C, Alfaro-Rodriguez MC, Muñoz J. Production of more sustainable emulsions formulated with eco-friendly materials. Journal of Cleaner Production. 2020;**243**:118661. DOI: 10.1016/j.jclepro.2019.118661

[57] Sunscreen Products Regulations in Europe [Internet]. 2024. Available from: https://taobe.consulting/european-regulations-sunscreen-products/ [Accessed: January 10, 2025]

[58] Suhail N, Alzahrani K, Basha J, Kizilbash N, et al. Microemulsion: Unique properties, pharmacological apllications, and targeted drug delivery. Frontiers in Nanotechnology. 2021;**3**:754889. DOI: 10.3389/fnano.2021.754889

[59] Xenakis A, Galani E, Papadimitriou V, Chatzidaki MD. Soft nanostructures for sun protection formulations. Current Opinion in Colloid & Interface Science. 2024;**71**:101803. DOI: 10.1016/j.cocis.2024.101803

[60] Chavda VP, Acharya D, Hala V, Daware S, Vora LK. Sunscreens: A comprehensive review with the application of nanotechnology. Journal of Drug Delivery Science and Technology. 2023;**86**:104720. DOI: 10.1016/j.jddst.2023.104720

[61] Reis-Mansur MCPP, Firmino Gomes CC, Nigro F, Ricci-Júnior E,

de Freitas ZMF, Dos Santos EP. Nanotechnology as a tool for optimizing topical photoprotective formulations containing Buriti oil (*Mauritia flexuosa*) and dry *Aloe vera* extracts: Stability and cytotoxicity evaluations. Pharmaceuticals (Basel). 2023;**16**(2):292. DOI: 10.3390/ph16020292

[62] Sanju N, Vineet M, Kumud M. Development and evaluation of a broad spectrum polyherbal sunscreen formulation using solid lipid nanoparticles of safranal. Journal of Cosmetic Dermatology. 2022;**21**(10): 4433-4446. DOI: 10.1111/jocd.14777

Chapter 7

Chemical Peels for Skin Rejuvenation and Anti-Aging in Darker Skin Tones

Nomakhosi Mpofana, Banathi Sihonqo, Mokgadi Ursula Makgobole, Celenkosini Thembelenkosini Nxumalo and Ncoza Cordelia Dlova

Abstract

Chemical peels are a popular skin care treatment that improves skin texture and a variety of skin concerns, including hyperpigmentation, acne scars, and signs of aging. While they can be effective for people with darker skin, their use requires careful consideration due to the unique properties of melanin-rich skin. People with darker skin types are more susceptible to hyperpigmentation and hypopigmentation; therefore, skin care specialists should tailor the treatments accordingly. Superficial peels, which frequently use alpha-hydroxy acids (AHAs) such as glycolic (GA) and lactic acid (LA), are mostly recommended for darker skin as they reduce the risk of post-inflammatory hyperpigmentation (PIH) and scarring. While chemical peels can provide significant benefits for skin rejuvenation in darker skin types, a tailored approach is required to ensure safety and efficacy. To mitigate possible risks, people are advised to seek treatment from experienced dermatologists or somatologists who understand the complexities of treating and managing darker skin. This book chapter examines the efficacy, benefits, and potential side effects of chemical peels in people with dark skin types. Ultimately, the goal is to improve understanding of how chemical peels can be used safely for skin rejuvenation in darker-skinned people.

Keywords: chemical peels, darker skin types, skin rejuvenation, safety, antiaging

1. Introduction

Chemical peels are a widely-used skincare procedure that enhances skin texture and tackles various dermatological issues, such as hyperpigmentation, acne scarring, and aging. While these treatments can be beneficial for individuals with darker complexions, their application necessitates careful consideration due to the distinct characteristics of melanin-rich skin. This summary explores the effectiveness, advantages, and potential risks associated with chemical peels for people with dark skin tones. The ultimate aim is to enhance our knowledge of how these cosmetic treatments can be safely employed for darker skin types, thus improving patient results and broadening dermatological treatment options. Mild peels, often utilizing alpha-hydroxy acids (AHAs) like glycolic and lactic acid, are typically suggested for darker skin to minimize the likelihood of post-inflammatory hyperpigmentation (PIH) and scarring. These treatments can enhance skin tone and texture while stimulating collagen production. However, individuals with darker skin are more prone to hyper- and hypopigmentation, necessitating tailored treatment approaches by skincare professionals. Common side effects include redness, swelling, and crusting, which may persist for varying durations depending on the peel depth. Additionally, some patients might experience acne outbreaks or infections without proper post-treatment care. Scarring is another concern, particularly with deeper peels. To reduce these potential risks, it is recommended that treatment be sought from experienced dermatologists or somatologists who are well-versed in the intricacies of treating and managing darker skin types. In summary, while chemical peels can offer significant skin rejuvenation benefits for individuals with darker complexions, a customized approach is essential to ensure both safety and efficacy.

2. The skin

The human body's largest organ, the skin, covers approximately 2 m^2 and acts as a protective shield against external threats, including physical, mechanical, chemical, and bacterial factors [1]. It also functions as a sensory organ, safeguards internal organs, and regulates moisture levels. The skin consists of three primary layers: epidermis, dermis, and hypodermis (also called subcutaneous tissue) [1]. As the most exposed organ, the skin displays signs of both environmental and chronological aging [2]. These manifestations include wrinkles, reduced firmness, and uneven pigmentation. Skin aging is a multifaceted biological process influenced by genetic factors, intrinsic aging, accumulated environmental damage, and extrinsic aging [3, 4]. These elements collectively lead to structural and physiological changes over time, occurring at varying but genetically predetermined rates [5]. Intrinsic or endogenous aging is typically associated with over time and is heavily influenced by genetics, cellular metabolism, hormones, and metabolic processes. In contrast, extrinsic or exogenous aging results from prolonged exposure to sunlight, pollution, and ionizing radiation, among other factors [3, 4]. Sun-exposed areas may experience roughness, elasticity loss, wrinkling, and pigmentary disorders, significantly impacting patients' quality of life and mental well-being [6]. The latter is often characterized by changes in melanocyte density, melanin concentration, or both, resulting in altered skin pigmentation (e.g., lentigos) [7]. Consequently, anti-aging products often incorporate depigmentation agents to address various signs of skin aging. The development of new anti-aging formulations has begun to focus on tackling both chronological and photoaging signs, including skin hyperpigmentation. Skin-lightening active ingredients can be derived from natural or synthetic sources and may act at different stages of the melanogenesis process.

3. The aging skin

The aging of the skin is a multifaceted process influenced by both endogenous and exogenous factors (**Figure 1**) that interact over time [8]. Natural aging leads

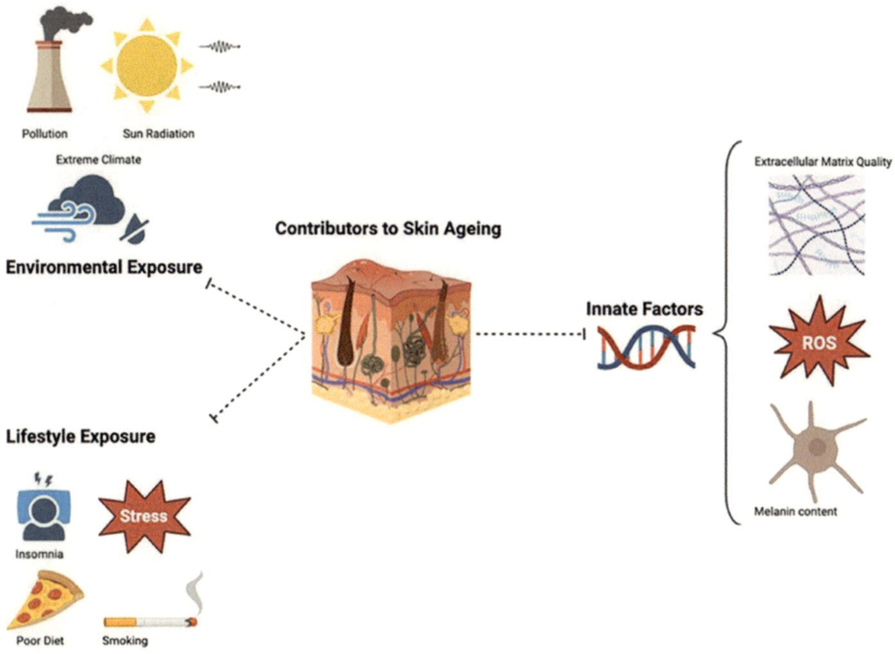

Figure 1.
An illustrated overview of factors contributing to the aging process of skin [8].

to decreased collagen synthesis, slower cellular regeneration, and reduced hydration, resulting in skin thinning, fine lines, and wrinkles [4]. External elements, especially environmental exposures such as ultraviolet radiation, atmospheric pollutants, and severe weather conditions, substantially expedite this progression [9]. For instance, ultraviolet (UV) exposure induces photoaging, leading to early-onset wrinkles, hyperpigmentation, and deterioration of skin texture. Personal habits also significantly impact skin health; for example, the use of tobacco constricts blood circulation, depriving the skin of essential nutrients, while suboptimal nutrition and insufficient rest hinder the skin's regenerative capabilities [8]. Collectively, these elements intensify the natural aging process, making the skin more susceptible to visible signs of aging and impacting its overall health and visual appearance.

3.1 Intrinsic aging

Intrinsic aging, also referred to as chronological aging, is an unavoidable, natural process governed by internal genetic factors [9]. This form of aging initiates in one's mid-twenties and progresses steadily, irrespective of external influences. Hallmarks of intrinsic aging include skin thinning, reduced collagen and elastin production, and a decelerated cellular turnover rate [4, 10]. These changes result in the emergence of fine lines and wrinkles and a decrease in skin firmness and elasticity. Moreover, intrinsic aging often leads to diminished skin hydration due to a reduction in natural oil production. While largely determined by an individual's genetic makeup, the effects of intrinsic aging are subtle and manifest over decades, making it a more gradual and predictable skin aging process [7].

3.2 Extrinsic aging

External environmental factors are responsible for extrinsic aging, which accelerates skin aging [11]. The primary contributor is ultraviolet (UV) radiation exposure, commonly known as photoaging [11, 12]. Additional factors include pollution, tobacco use, inadequate nutrition, chronic stress, and repetitive facial expressions. In contrast to intrinsic aging, extrinsic aging can vary considerably based on lifestyle choices and environmental conditions [1, 11]. Its effects typically manifest as uneven skin tone, pronounced wrinkles, hyperpigmentation, and a coarse, leathery texture. The rapid breakdown of collagen and elastin fibers is largely attributed to free radical damage caused by UV rays and pollution. Extrinsic aging can often be prevented or mitigated through protective measures such as sunscreen application, maintaining a healthy lifestyle, and adopting effective skincare routines [10].

4. Determination of aging

To evaluate and quantify the visible effects of intrinsic and extrinsic aging, various clinical scales have been developed. These standardized methods consider factors such as wrinkles, sagging, pigmentation, and overall skin texture to guide treatment strategies and monitor the effectiveness of interventions.

- *Glogau classification of photoaging*: This scale divides photoaging into four grades based on clinical features, including wrinkles, pigmentation, and the necessity for makeup to conceal imperfections. It is commonly used to assess the severity of sun-induced damage [13, 14].

- *Fitzpatrick wrinkle classification system*: This system evaluates the depth and extent of facial wrinkles, focusing on specific areas like the forehead, eyes, and nasolabial folds. It aids in determining suitable anti-aging treatments, such as chemical peels or injectables [15].

- *Global Facial Wrinkle Scale (GFWS)*: A comprehensive tool that assesses wrinkles across the entire face, offering an objective evaluation of the severity and distribution of aging signs [13].

- *D'Alexis scale*: Designed for individuals with darker skin tones, this scale concentrates on pigmentation issues, such as hyperpigmentation and post-inflammatory discolorations that are prevalent with aging in melanin-rich skin [15].

5. Understanding chemical peels

Dermatological treatments known as chemical peels involve applying exfoliating agents to remove damaged skin layers, encouraging the growth of healthier, more even, and luminous skin. These procedures are classified into superficial, medium, and deep peels, depending on how deeply they penetrate and the specific acids utilized, such as alpha-hydroxy acids (AHAs), beta-hydroxy acids (BHAs), and trichloroacetic acid (TCA). Chemical peels primarily aim to tackle various skin issues, including rough texture, dark spots, acne scarring, and aging signs. By boosting skin cell renewal and collagen synthesis, these treatments not only enhance skin appearance but also improve its underlying structure, providing both esthetic and therapeutic advantages.

Chemical peels are minimally invasive dermatological solutions created to exfoliate the skin and promote natural regeneration [2]. This is accomplished by applying a chemical mixture to the skin, causing controlled injury to the epidermis or deeper layers, based on the peel type. The damaged skin eventually sloughs off, unveiling a smoother, more uniform, and revitalized skin layer beneath [16]. The main objective of chemical peels is to enhance skin appearance and health by addressing concerns such as uneven texture, hyperpigmentation, wrinkles, acne scars, and sun damage [2, 17]. Furthermore, chemical peels can improve skin elasticity and stimulate collagen production, making them an effective treatment for aging symptoms [18]. Customized formulations allow for a broad range of applications, making chemical peels suitable for diverse skin types and conditions.

5.1 Categories of chemical peels

Chemical peels are classified as superficial, medium, and deep peels (**Table 1**), each designed to address particular skin issues and degrees of aging [20]. These treatments function by removing layers of skin, stimulating cellular regeneration, and improving overall skin texture and appearance.

5.1.1 Superficial peels

Superficial peels represent the gentlest form of chemical exfoliation, targeting the skin's outermost layer and epidermis [20]. Typically formulated with alpha-hydroxy acids (AHAs), like glycolic acid, or beta-hydroxy acids (BHAs), such as salicylic acid, these peels are suitable for treating minor aging signs, including fine lines, uneven

Very superficial	Superficial	Medium	Deep
1. Alpha-hydroxy acids (AHAs) • Mandelic acid (MA) • Glycolic acid: 20–70% (GA) 2. Beta-hydroxy acids (BHAs) • Salicylic acid: 20–30% 3. Poly-hydroxy acids (PHAs) • Gluconolactone 4. Bionic acids (BAs) • Lactobionic acid • Maltobionic acid Aromatic hydroxy acids (AMAs)	Trichloroacetic acid (TCA): 20–35% GA: 70% Jessner's solution	TCA: 50% Monheit's combination Jessner's solution and 35% TCA Coleman's combination (70% GA and 35% TCA)	Phenol: 80% Baker-Gordon phenolic peeling: 25–50% phenol and croton oil

Table 1.
Categories of chemical peels based on their level of skin penetration [19].

skin tone, and slight roughness [21]. They also boost hydration, leaving the skin refreshed and glowing, with minimal recovery time. Superficial peels are a popular option for individuals seeking gradual improvement through regular treatments.

5.1.2 Medium peels

Chemical peels of medium depth extend into the upper layers of the dermis [22]. These treatments commonly utilize trichloroacetic acid (TCA) or higher concentrations of alpha-hydroxy acids (AHAs) to target more noticeable signs of aging, including moderate wrinkles, sun-induced damage, and discoloration issues [23]. Medium-depth peels enhance collagen production and facilitate substantial skin renewal, leading to a more youthful and even complexion. The recovery process for these peels involves skin shedding and redness lasting several days, making them ideal for individuals seeking visible improvements without resorting to deeper peeling treatments [16, 20]. These peels are particularly suited for clients who desire noticeable results but prefer to avoid more intensive procedures.

5.1.3 Deep peels

For advanced signs of aging, the most intensive treatment available is deep chemical peels [19, 21]. These procedures target the lower dermis using high-strength TCA or phenol solutions to address severe wrinkles, extensive sun damage, and major pigmentation issues (**Figure 2**). By promoting collagen production and skin remodeling, these peels produce significant and enduring results [19]. However, they require a substantial recovery period, often necessitating several weeks of downtime and

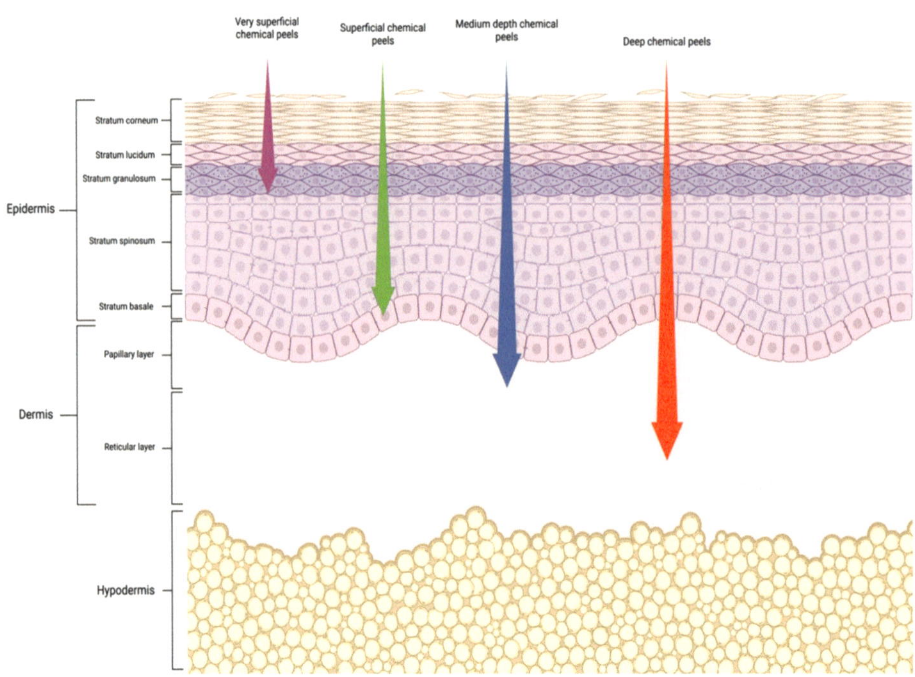

Figure 2.
Chemical peel penetration depth [19].

careful post-treatment management. Typically administered by healthcare professionals, deep peels are recommended for individuals with extensive aging concerns or skin damage.

6. Mechanism of action: Exfoliation and skin rejuvenation

The effectiveness of chemical peels stems from two main processes: exfoliation and skin renewal, which contribute to enhancing the look and condition of mature skin [24]. These mechanisms promote the natural regeneration of skin cells and improve the overall quality of the skin.

6.1 Exfoliation and skin renewal

Chemical peels contain active components that break down the connections between dead cells in the skin's outermost layer, known as the stratum corneum [24, 25]. This process of controlled exfoliation eliminates dull and damaged skin, exposing fresher, healthier layers beneath. While superficial peels generally affect the epidermis, medium and deep peels can reach the dermis, depending on their chemical makeup and strength [22]. The exfoliation process enhances skin texture, tone, and clarity by removing accumulated debris and dead cells. Additionally, it facilitates better absorption of active skincare ingredients, thus enhancing their effectiveness. Skin texture can be enhanced through chemical peels, which work by removing the top layer of skin (stratum corneum) and promoting the growth of a more refined epidermis [26, 27]. Alpha-hydroxy acids (AHAs), including glycolic and lactic acids, improve skin smoothness and even out skin tone by dissolving the bonds between keratinocytes [26]. This action helps diminish discoloration, tackle surface flaws, and bring back skin radiance. Research indicates that light peels are particularly beneficial for boosting skin luminosity and tactile smoothness, making them well-suited for those with minor texture concerns [18, 25]. These treatments effectively reduce roughness and address uneven skin tone, resulting in a more polished appearance.

7. Benefits of chemical peels for skin rejuvenation

Chemical peels enhance skin renewal by promoting cellular regeneration and natural repair mechanisms [25, 28]. This process is facilitated through the activation of fibroblasts, which generate essential structural proteins like collagen and elastin, crucial for maintaining skin's firmness and flexibility. Specifically, medium and deep peels induce an inflammatory response within the dermis, stimulating the production of new collagen and glycosaminoglycans, which contribute to improved skin hydration and fullness [25]. With continued use, these treatments can diminish the appearance of fine lines, wrinkles, uneven pigmentation, and other age-related skin concerns. The dual benefits of exfoliation and skin rejuvenation make chemical peels an effective method for enhancing skin health and restoring a more youthful appearance [18]. By eliminating damaged skin layers and encouraging the growth of new, healthy cells, chemical peels can effectively counteract visible signs of aging and environmental damage.

In the field of dermatology, chemical peels have emerged as a crucial technique for skin revitalization [18]. According to Rostkowska et al. [5], these treatments employ exfoliating substances, including alpha-hydroxy acids (AHAs), beta-hydroxy acids (BHAs), and trichloroacetic acid (TCA), to promote skin cell regeneration, enhance skin texture, and tackle various dermatological issues. The beneficial effects of chemical peels are attributed to several processes: the removal of surface skin cells, the activation of fibroblasts in the dermis, and the acceleration of keratinocyte production. These mechanisms collectively result in a more refreshed and younger-looking complexion [26].

7.1 Reduction of hyperpigmentation and dark spots

Chemical peels are frequently used to address hyperpigmentation issues, including melasma, post-inflammatory hyperpigmentation (PIH), and age spots [29]. Alpha-hydroxy acids (AHAs) effectively diminish hyperpigmentation by enhancing the shedding of pigmented skin cells and suppressing tyrosinase, an essential enzyme in melanin production. For example, glycolic acid deeply penetrates the skin's outer layer, helping to diminish dark spots and create a more uniform complexion [30]. Peels of moderate depth, which combine trichloroacetic acid (TCA) with AHAs, have demonstrated effectiveness in treating more stubborn pigmentation disorders [22]. Furthermore, the application of sonophoresis to enhance the absorption of peeling agents can boost treatment efficacy, particularly for individuals with darker skin tones who are more susceptible to PIH.

7.2 Stimulation of collagen production for antiaging effects

Chemical peels enhance the production of collagen, a crucial element for maintaining youthful and firm skin. Alpha-hydroxy acids (AHAs), particularly glycolic acid, activate dermal fibroblasts, resulting in increased synthesis of collagen and glycosaminoglycans [4, 20]. This process improves the skin's structural integrity and elasticity, thereby diminishing the visibility of fine lines and wrinkles. While deeper peels require longer recovery periods, they are especially beneficial for treating advanced aging signs, such as prominent wrinkles and skin laxity [4]. These treatments can reverse the structural damage caused by intrinsic and photoaging by promoting dermal remodeling. The addition of antioxidant-rich formulations to the peel further enhanced collagen production by reducing oxidative stress.

8. Treatment considerations for darker skin tones

When treating aging skin in individuals with darker complexions, it is crucial to exercise caution and thoughtfulness to achieve safe and effective results. The high melanin content in darker skin types poses distinct challenges that require specialized strategies and a thorough understanding of the skin's biological responses [31]. These unique characteristics necessitate a customized approach to ensure optimal treatment outcomes. Individuals with darker complexions face a higher risk of complications from chemical peel treatments, both during and after the procedure [31]. The primary concern is the increased likelihood of developing post-inflammatory hyperpigmentation (PIH), a condition where the skin overproduces melanin in reaction to trauma or irritation, causing dark patches to appear [31, 32]. Furthermore, these individuals may experience hypopigmentation (lighter skin areas) and keloid formation, especially if the treatment affects deeper skin layers. Moreover, the uneven distribution of melanin can result in inconsistent outcomes if the treatment process is not carefully monitored and managed.

9. Importance of tailored formulations and concentrations

For darker skin tones, specialized formulations and concentrations play a crucial role in reducing risks and obtaining desired outcomes. Gentle, surface-level peels utilizing alpha-hydroxy acids (AHAs), such as lactic acid, or beta-hydroxy acids (BHAs), like salicylic acid, are typically safer choices due to their mild exfoliating properties [24]. Under professional guidance, medium-depth peels, including trichloroacetic acid (TCA) at lower concentrations, can be applied with caution [22]. The risk of hyperpigmentation can be further mitigated through customized pre-treatment protocols, which may involve the use of melanin-regulating agents like hydroquinone or azelaic acid to control melanin production before the procedure.

10. Role of melanin in skin response to chemical peels

In individuals with darker skin tones, melanin serves as a crucial factor in determining the skin's reaction to chemical substances [31]. According to Mar et al. [17], this natural pigment not only shields against ultraviolet radiation but also affects the skin's healing processes. Chemical exfoliation procedures can cause irritation or inflammation, potentially leading to excessive stimulation of melanocytes, the cells responsible for melanin production [24]. This overstimulation may result in uneven skin coloration. The extent to which the chemical penetrates the skin is also significant; deeper chemical peels are more likely to disrupt the distribution of melanin, potentially causing irregularities in pigmentation [19]. By comprehending these mechanisms, skincare professionals can make informed decisions regarding treatment methods and techniques to achieve optimal results for patients with darker complexions.

11. Safety and efficacy

11.1 Recommended types of chemical peels for darker skin

Due to their mild nature and lower likelihood of causing post-inflammatory hyperpigmentation (PIH), specific chemical peel varieties are especially appropriate for individuals with darker skin complexions [20]. For addressing skin aging issues such as fine lines, hyperpigmentation, and uneven texture, chemical peels can offer a safe and effective treatment option [25]. However, to achieve the best outcomes, especially for those with darker complexions, it is crucial to carefully choose the appropriate peel type, ensure professional application, and strictly follow pre-treatment and post-treatment care instructions.

Glycolic acid: Sugarcane-derived glycolic acid, a type of alpha-hydroxy acid (AHA), is an effective ingredient for superficial peeling treatments [33]. When applied in small amounts, it provides gentle exfoliation, enhances skin texture, and diminishes the visibility of wrinkles. Additionally, using AHA in low concentrations helps minimize the risk of skin discoloration.

Salicylic acid: Salicylic acid, an oil-soluble compound known as beta-hydroxy acid (BHA), is particularly effective for people with darker complexions and skin that is prone to oiliness or acne. This substance effectively clears pores, alleviates inflammation, and assists in addressing pigmentation issues [17].

Lactic acid: Originating from milk, lactic acid is a gentle alpha-hydroxy acid (AHA) that moisturizes and gently removes dead skin cells [34]. This makes it a suitable choice for individuals with sensitive skin or darker complexions.

Mandelic acid: Mandelic acid, a larger molecular AHA, is exceptionally mild and effective in addressing pigmentation concerns while minimizing the potential for skin irritation [30].

11.2 Importance of professional administration by trained dermatologists

The efficacy and safety of chemical peels are largely contingent on their application by skilled practitioners, especially for medium and deep treatments. Dermatologists and certified skin care specialists must have the following crucial competencies [5, 19]:

- Precise evaluation of a patient's skin condition and issues.
- Determination of the most suitable peel formulation, strength, and application time.
- Observation of skin reactions during the procedure to avoid excessive exfoliation or injury.
- Prompt intervention in case of unfavorable responses. Expert administration minimizes the risk of complications and guarantees a secure and productive treatment outcome.

12. The importance of pre-treatment and post-treatment care to minimize risks

To maximize effectiveness and minimize potential issues, thorough pre- and post-treatment care is crucial when undergoing chemical peels [35].

- *Pre-treatment care:* Refrain from exposing skin to sunlight and using tanning methods for a minimum of 2 weeks before the treatment. To mitigate post-inflammatory hyperpigmentation (PIH), substances that regulate melanin production, including hydroquinone and kojic acid, were utilized. Products containing exfoliants and retinoids were stopped 3–5 days before the procedure. A preliminary test was conducted to evaluate the skin's response to the chemical peel solution.
- *Post-treatment care:* To shield the skin from ultraviolet radiation, a high-protection sunscreen (SPF 30+) should be applied each day. Mild, moisturizing skincare products should be used to calm the skin and combat dehydration. For a minimum of 7 days, abrasive products like exfoliants or retinoids should be avoided.

13. Alternative treatments

For individuals with darker complexions, there are effective and safe alternatives to chemical peels when addressing aging skin or other concerns. These alternative methods (**Table 2**) typically focus on similar issues, including hyperpigmentation,

Treatment	Mechanism	Safety	Efficacy
Microneedling:	The process involves creating controlled micro-injuries in the skin using thin needles, which prompts the production of collagen and elastin.	This method is particularly safe for individuals with darker skin tones, as it does not use heat and minimizes the risk of post-inflammatory hyperpigmentation (PIH).	It effectively enhances skin texture, diminishes fine lines, and lightens hyperpigmentation. The application of growth factors or vitamin C serum during the procedure often amplifies the results.
Laser treatments	Lasers, including Nd: YAG and fractional non-ablative types, address specific skin issues like pigmentation, texture, and wrinkles by delivering concentrated energy to promote skin regeneration.	With proper laser selection and settings, the treatment is safe for darker skin tones. However, caution is necessary to avoid excessive heat that may trigger changes in pigmentation.	Lasers offer precise targeting of specific concerns, such as dark spots or deep wrinkles, and typically yield quicker results compared to chemical peels.
Microdermabrasion	This method employs a dedicated device to exfoliate the skin's outer layer, resulting in a smoother and more radiant complexion.	It is a non-invasive procedure that is safe for darker skin tones when performed gently to prevent irritation.	While suitable for addressing mild skin issues like dullness and surface-level pigmentation, it is less effective for deeper concerns compared to peels or lasers.

Table 2.
Comparison of alternative treatments with other cosmetic procedures safe for darker skin [10, 36].

wrinkles, and skin texture irregularities. Furthermore, combining these alternative treatments with chemical peels can lead to improved outcomes through a complementary approach [10, 36].

14. Synergistic effects when combined with chemical peels

Integrating chemical peels with other skin care procedures can enhance outcomes by targeting multiple skin issues simultaneously [36].

Chemical peels and microneedling: Applying a chemical peel following microneedling improves the absorption of active components, enhancing skin renewal [37]. This approach is especially beneficial for treating acne scars, discoloration, and rough skin texture. Proper timing is essential; experts typically schedule treatments several weeks apart to ensure adequate healing and prevent overstimulation.

Chemical peeling and laser treatment: Mild chemical peels can be utilized to ready the skin for laser procedures by eliminating surface debris and maximizing laser penetration. Peels performed after laser treatments can help sustain results by addressing remaining pigmentation or fine lines [36]. Careful planning of this combination is necessary to minimize the risk of excessive skin irritation or inflammation.

Chemical peels and topical treatments: Chemical peels improve the skin's ability to absorb active ingredients found in skincare products like retinoids, antioxidants, and hydroquinone [38]. This combination optimizes results while preserving skin health.

15. Patient education and expectations

15.1 Setting realistic goals for treatment outcomes

When exploring chemical peels as a method for skin renewal, particularly for those with darker complexions, it is crucial to manage expectations appropriately. The main advantages of these treatments include enhanced skin texture, more uniform skin tone, and a decrease in issues like hyperpigmentation, acne scarring, and aging indicators. However, it is important to note that these improvements may not be immediate and could require several sessions to achieve the best results. For individuals with darker skin tones, mild peels, typically containing alpha-hydroxy acids (AHAs) such as glycolic or lactic acid, are often suggested. These treatments are generally successful in enhancing skin tone and boosting collagen production while minimizing the risk of complications like post-inflammatory hyperpigmentation (PIH). Nevertheless, it is essential to recognize that while treatment can lead to substantial improvements, outcomes may differ based on individual skin reactions and the extent of existing skin issues. Patients should be informed about the gradual nature of the process. They need to understand that while chemical peels can enhance skin appearance, they may not provide an immediate or dramatic change. To maintain the results, ongoing maintenance treatments and proper skin care routines following the peel are essential.

15.2 Understanding potential side effects and recovery time

As with any esthetic treatment, chemical peels come with potential risks, and patients should be aware of these possible side effects. Common reactions include redness, swelling, and crusting, which are more pronounced with deeper peels. Superficial peels generally have quicker recovery periods. Individuals with darker complexions face an increased likelihood of hyperpigmentation or hypopigmentation, especially if post-treatment instructions are not strictly adhered to. The duration of recovery is contingent on the depth of the peel. Superficial treatments may result in minimal downtime, with patients typically experiencing mild redness or flaking that subsides within a few days. More intense peels necessitate longer recovery periods, spanning from several days to a few weeks. The risk of complications, such as scarring and acne outbreaks, may be heightened if proper aftercare is not followed. To minimize risks, it is recommended that patients seek treatment from skilled dermatologists or skin experts who are well-versed in managing darker skin types. Patients should also be educated about the importance of sun protection, avoiding harsh chemicals, and following a gentle skincare regimen to promote healing. In the end, well-informed patients are better positioned to manage their expectations, follow aftercare guidelines, and achieve optimal results from their chemical peel treatment.

15.3 Importance of follow-up consultations for optimal results

Post-treatment consultations are essential for optimizing the outcomes of chemical peels, especially for individuals with darker complexions [31]. These follow-up sessions enable healthcare professionals to evaluate the skin's reaction, tackle any issues, and modify the treatment strategy as needed. For patients with darker skin tones, subsequent visits are vital for monitoring potential complications like hyperpigmentation or scarring, which may necessitate adjustments to the treatment protocol. During these appointments, medical practitioners can evaluate the healing process, offer advice on skincare and sun protection, and confirm that the skin is responding as anticipated. Moreover, these follow-up meetings allow the practitioner to assess whether further treatments are required to achieve the desired results. Given that multiple peels may be necessary for optimal skin rejuvenation, regular follow-ups ensure that the treatment plan is customized to meet the individual's specific needs and that the desired outcomes are attained safely and effectively.

16. Conclusion

For individuals with darker complexions, customized chemical peels can provide substantial advantages in skin renewal. These treatments enhance skin texture, tackle discoloration issues, and diminish the visibility of acne marks and aging indicators. Gentle peels, particularly those utilizing AHAs, are especially appropriate for darker skin tones; hence, they minimize the potential for complications like post-inflammatory hyperpigmentation while encouraging collagen formation and promoting a more uniform skin appearance. Despite the effectiveness of chemical peels, those with darker skin must consult experienced dermatologists or somatologists, as they are well-trained in treating melanin-rich complexions. These professionals can create tailored treatment strategies that address each patient's specific skin concern and reduce the likelihood of adverse effects. By collaborating with a competent practitioner and adhering to a personalized regimen, patients can safely and effectively achieve optimal outcomes.

Conflict of interest

The authors declare no conflict of interest.

Author details

Nomakhosi Mpofana[1*], Banathi Sihonqo[1], Mokgadi Ursula Makgobole[1], Celenkosini Thembelenkosini Nxumalo[2,3] and Ncoza Cordelia Dlova[4]

1 Department of Somatology, Durban University of Technology—Ritson Campus, Durban, KwaZulu-Natal, South Africa

2 Office of the DVC Research and Innovation, University of the Western Cape, Bellville, Western Cape, South Africa

3 Discipline of Nursing, School of Nursing and Public Health, University of KwaZulu-Natal, Durban, South Africa

4 Dermatology Department, Nelson R. Mandela School of Medicine, University of KwaZulu-Natal, Durban, South Africa

*Address all correspondence to: nomakhosim@dut.ac.za

References

[1] Tobin DJ. Introduction to skin aging. Journal of Tissue Viability. 2017;**26**(1):37-46

[2] Jiang X, Li X. Chemical peels for skin rejuvenation. In: Skin Photoaging (Second Edition). Bristol, UK: IOP Publishing; 2024. pp. 6-1-6-22

[3] Hussein RS et al. Influences on skin and intrinsic aging: Biological, environmental, and therapeutic insights. Journal of Cosmetic Dermatology. 2025;**24**(2):e16688

[4] Mohiuddin AK. Skin aging & modern age anti-aging strategies. International Journal of Clinical Dermatology & Research. 2019;**7**:209-240

[5] Rostkowska E et al. Dermatological management of aged skin. Cosmetics. 2023;**10**(2):55

[6] Griffiths T. Facial ageing: How do we measure up? British Journal of Dermatology. 2015;**172**(5):1180-1195

[7] Dobos G et al. Evaluation of skin ageing: A systematic review of clinical scales. British Journal of Dermatology. 2015;**172**(5):1249-1261

[8] Tao BK et al. Periocular aging across populations and esthetic considerations: A narrative review. Journal of Clinical Medicine. 2025;**14**(2):535

[9] Farage M et al. Intrinsic and extrinsic factors in skin ageing: A review. International Journal of Cosmetic Science. 2008;**30**(2):87-95

[10] Gangwar A, Sharma V, Sharma R. Combinational treatment approaches for acanthosis nigricans: A review. Archives of Dermatological Research. 2025;**317**(1):179

[11] Krutmann J et al. Environmentally-induced (extrinsic) skin aging: Exposomal factors and underlying mechanisms. Journal of Investigative Dermatology. 2021;**141**(4):1096-1103

[12] Fang JY et al. Skin aging caused by intrinsic or extrinsic processes characterized with functional proteomics. Proteomics. 2016;**16**(20):2718-2731

[13] Oesch S et al. A correlation of the Glogau scale with VISIA-CR complexion analysis measurements in assessing facial photoaging for clinical research. Aesthetic Surgery Journal. 2022;**42**(10):1175-1184

[14] Sukma PMG et al. Photoaging assessment by Glogau classification: Correlation of dermoscopy findings in the coastal population of Indonesia. Acta Dermatovenerologica Alpina, Pannonica et Adriatica. 2024;**33**(1):1-5

[15] Kappes U. Skin ageing and wrinkles: Clinical and photographic scoring. Journal of Cosmetic Dermatology. 2004;**3**(1):23-25

[16] Landau M, Bageorgeou F. Update on chemical peels. Dermatologic Clinics. 2024;**42**(1):13-20

[17] Mar K et al. Treatment of post-inflammatory hyperpigmentation in skin of colour: A systematic review. Journal of Cutaneous Medicine and Surgery. 2024;**28**(5):473-480

[18] Patole SP, Naikawadi ND, Redasani V. Revitalize your skin: A comprehensive review of chemical peel. Asian Journal of Pharmaceutical Research and Development. 2024;**11**(3):94-101

[19] Sołdacka D, Barańska-Rybak W. Evaluation of safety and efficacy of chemical peels with and without sonophoresis on selected skin parameters—A prospective comparative study. Cosmetics. 2024;**11**(6):185. ISSN:2079-9284

[20] Lee KC et al. Basic chemical peeling: Superficial and medium-depth peels. Journal of the American Academy of Dermatology. 2019;**81**(2):313-324

[21] Tang S-C, Yang J-H. Dual effects of alpha-hydroxy acids on the skin. Molecules. 2018;**23**(4):863

[22] Kumari R, Thappa DM. Comparative study of trichloroacetic acid versus glycolic acid chemical peels in the treatment of melasma. Indian Journal of Dermatology, Venereology and Leprology. 2010;**76**:447

[23] Kubiak M, Mucha P, Rotsztejn H. Comparative study of 15% trichloroacetic acid peel combined with 70% glycolic acid and 35% trichloroacetic acid peel for the treatment of photodamaged facial skin in aging women. Journal of Cosmetic Dermatology. 2020;**19**(1):137-146

[24] Doktorova Z et al. Skin exfoliation: Indications, contraindications, and side effects. Varna Medical Forum. 2024;**13**(1):120-133

[25] Pathak A, Mohan R, Rohrich RJ. Chemical peels: Role of chemical peels in facial rejuvenation today. Plastic and Reconstructive Surgery. 2020;**145**(1):58e-66e

[26] Wisniewski JD, Ellis DL, Lupo MP. Facial rejuvenation: Combining cosmeceuticals with cosmetic procedures. Cutis. 2014;**94**(3):122-126

[27] Haney B. Superficial chemical peels. In: Aesthetic Procedures: Nurse Practitioner's Guide to Cosmetic Dermatology. Los Angeles, USA: Springer; 2024. pp. 79-86

[28] Obagi S. Chemical Peels: Procedures and Complications. Walth Mass: UpToDate; 2020

[29] Agbai ON, Quiñonez RL, Taylor SC. Postinflammatory hyperpigmentation: Treatment and prevention. In: Cosmetic Procedures in Skin of Color. Philadelphia, PA: Elsevier; 2025. pp. 105-124

[30] Jeon H et al. Enhancement of exfoliating effects through the novel cosmetic ingredient mandelic acid_carnitine ion-pairing complex. Skin Research and Technology. 2024;**30**(6):e13788

[31] Harnchoowong S, Vachiramon V, Jurairattanaporn N. Cosmetic considerations in dark-skinned patients. Clinical, Cosmetic and Investigational Dermatology. 2024;**17**:259-277

[32] Jiryis B et al. Management of melasma: Laser and other therapies—Review study. Journal of Clinical Medicine. 2024;**13**(5):1468

[33] Seleteng-Kose LE, Likoetla P, Motjotji L. Plants of commercial importance in Lesotho: Ethnobotanical and pharmacological insights. Cosmetics. 2023;**10**(1):28

[34] Karwal K, Mukovozov I. Topical AHA in dermatology: Formulations, mechanisms of action, efficacy, and future perspectives. Cosmetics. 2023;**10**(5):131

[35] Almeman AA. Evaluating the efficacy and safety of alpha-hydroxy acids in dermatological practice: A comprehensive clinical and legal review. Clinical, Cosmetic and

Investigational Dermatology. 2024;**17**:1661-1685

[36] Been MJ, Mangat DS. Laser and face peel procedures in non-Caucasians. Facial Plastic Surgery Clinics. 2014;**22**(3):447-452

[37] Lee JC, Daniels MA, Roth MZ. Mesotherapy, microneedling, and chemical peels. Clinics in Plastic Surgery. 2016;**43**(3):583-595

[38] Grimes PE. Chemical peels: Nuances and best practices for skin of color. In: Cosmetic Procedures in Skin of Color. Philadelphia, PA: Elsevier; 2025. pp. 169-180

Chapter 8

Trending Topical Ingredients for Hyperpigmentation

Özlem Karadağ Köse

Abstract

With the increase in social media usage today, there is a desire to achieve a completely perfect, smooth, and filtered appearance of the skin. As the demand for bright, smooth, spot-free, and poreless skin rises, the application of topical products and the search for using new ingredients are escalating. It is believed that skin aging plays a role in all types of hyperpigmentation, including uneven skin tone, post-inflammatory hyperpigmentation (PIH), melasma, and any combination of these. Hydroquinone is the effective first-line treatment choice and has been used for many years, but its use has decreased in recent years due to side effects. Lately, the role of retinoic acid derivatives in skin aging and hyperpigmentation treatment has been identified, and new retinoic acid derivatives are especially used in PIH. Niacinamide, a type of vitamin B, and ascorbic acid, a vitamin C derivative, are notable molecules. In addition to the many antioxidants that have emerged, plant-derived substances have also come to the forefront in topical treatments in recent years due to their minimal side effects and similar results to hydroquinone. This article summarizes the trending topical ingredients in the treatment of hyperpigmentation.

Keywords: hyperpigmentation, melasma, spots, trend ingredients, treatment

1. Introduction

Hyperpigmentation is one of the most common skin disorders. While there are many conditions that cause hyperpigmentation, melasma and post-inflammatory hyperpigmentation, along with acne, freckles, lentigo, and photoaging, are the most prominent. Ultraviolet and visible light increase the hyperpigmentation. There are 14 organic and 2 inorganic (zinc oxide, titanium dioxide) FDA-approved filters [1]. It is recommended that all patients, including Fitzpatrick skin phototype IV-VI, use a broad-spectrum tinted SPF of ≥30 daily [2]. However, broad-spectrum sunscreens are not protective against UVA and visible light (VL), which causes hyperpigmentation. Sunscreens containing iron oxide have been shown to be very effective in protecting against visible light [2]. In addition of certain supporting antioxidants such as vitamin C, E, licochalcone A, and diethylhexyl syringylidenemalonate to sunscreens for the removal of the radicals and prevention of lipid peroxidation is also a new trend in sunscreens [3]. More clinical research is needed regarding the use of antioxidants in sunscreen products.

Hydroquinone has been proposed as the gold standard treatment for melasma for many years. Studies conducted since the 1950s have shown a 60–90% regression in

IntechOpen

pigmentation within 5–7 weeks of use in a range of 2–4% [4]. Its usage is declining due to the numerous side effects, including contact dermatitis and exogenous ochronosis. In 2006, high-dose hydroquinone use in animals was found to be carcinogenic [4]. In 2020, over-the-counter use was banned by CARES, and products that have since received FDA approval post-2020 are being sold by prescription in the U.S. The triple combination cream known as the Willis formula contains hydroquinone and tretinoin, which have also been found effective; however, the long-term use is limited due to the side effects of its ingredients [4].

This article aims to summarize the hyperpigmentation treatments, especially those trending in recent years, apart from hydroquinone.

2. Trending topical ingredients for hyperpigmentation

2.1 Ascorbic acid (vitamin C)

Vitamin C, also known as ascorbic acid (AA) and its derivatives (ascorbyl-6 palmitate, magnesium ascorbyl phosphate), is used in the treatment of hyperpigmentation at varying percentages between 5 and 20% [1]. Vitamin C is a hydrophilic antioxidant, inhibiting tyrosinase and stimulating collagen synthesis. It is suitable for both day and night use, helping sunscreens remain on the epidermis longer. It has been found that topical vitamin C exhibits a synergistic effect with topical vitamins E and A. Generally, vitamin C is a molecule that is difficult to stabilize and penetrate [1].

In a study with 16 patients comparing topical 5% AA and 4% hydroquinone, an earlier response was found with hydroquinone, while no differences in efficacy were observed by the 4th month [5]. In another study involving 39 patients, a significant decrease in melanin area and severity index (MASI) was observed with 25% AA after 16 weeks [6].

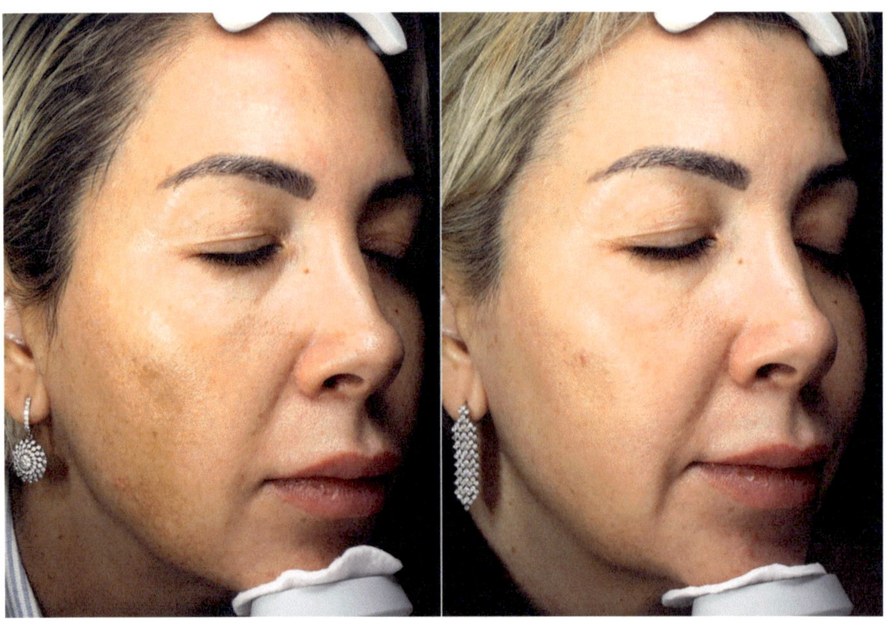

Figure 1.
Sunscreen (SPF50 + VL), ascorbic acid 2 times/day, and azelaic acid once/day.

When considering the side effects of topical vitamin C, it has generally been found to be well tolerated. However, high concentrations like 25% have been associated with irritation, erythema, and burning (**Figure 1**) [6].

2.2 Niacinamide

Niacinamide is the biologically active form of vitamin B3, also known as niacin. Niacinamide is a precursor to the nicotinamide adenine dinucleotide molecule [7]. It is most commonly found in yeast and root vegetables. Niacinamide is often present in creams at concentrations ranging from 2–5% [7]. When we look at the mechanism of action of niacinamide, we see that it prevents the transfer of melanosomes to keratinocytes. Niacinamide is also effective in reducing melanogenesis [8]. Additionally, niacinamide is an anti-inflammatory molecule, and it reduces solar degenerative changes. Due to these properties, it has become a preferred option in topical treatments that have gained popularity in recent years for hyperpigmentation [8].

Looking at the studies conducted with niacinamide, there was no significant difference in MASI scores when comparing creams containing 4% hydroquinone and 4% niacinamide in 27 patients with melasma [9]. Both treatments resulted in a significant decrease in MASI scores and have been reported as effective treatments [9]. In another study on spot treatment with niacinamide, the comparison between 4% niacinamide and 0.05% all-trans retinoic acid (ATRA) found that niacinamide was more effective than ATRA [10]. Niacinamide has been reported to be effective against different forms of hyperpigmentation, including axillary and post-inflammatory forms and hyperpigmentation that is triggered by ultraviolet and blue light [8].

It is considered a safe option for hyperpigmentation removal. More studies are necessary to demonstrate its efficacy as a standalone spot treatment.

2.3 Tranexamic acid

Tranexamic acid has been used as an antifibrinolytic in severe bleeding. It prevents the binding of plasminogen to keratinocytes and inhibits the ultraviolet-induced plasminogen activator and keratinocytes [11]. Tranexamic acid reduces melanogenic factors such as prostaglandins, leukotrienes, fibroblast growth factor, α-melanocyte stimulating hormone, and arachidonic acid. Likewise, tranexamic acid also contributes to a reduction in CD 31+ blood vessels and endothelin. Meanwhile, it acts as a tyrosinase inhibitor [12].

Research conducted with tranexamic acid indicates that more studies on melasma and PIH are needed. These publications on tranexamic acid have shown that it could potentially be an effective therapeutic agent for treating hyperpigmentation. Topical tranexamic acid has been used in liposomal form in a ratio of 2–5% over a period of 2–3 months in a study involving 39 patients. When comparing 3% tranexamic acid with 3% hydroquinone and 0.1% dexamethasone used together, no significant difference in efficacy was found between the two groups [13, 14]. In another study with 60 patients comparing 5% tranexamic acid and 2% hydroquinone, a significant lightening effect was observed in both groups by the end of the 12 weeks, with no meaningful difference between the two groups [15]. Furthermore, in another split-face research using topical tranexamic acid, 5% tranexamic acid was used on one side of the face, while 4% hydroquinone was used on the other side [16]. Similarly, a notable equal lightening effect was observed on both sides, with no difference in potency [16].

Tranexamic acid is a well-tolerated molecule in general.

2.4 Retinoic acid

Vitamin A analogs are used for treating acne and related PIH, as well as melasma, lentigo, and photoaging [17]. Retinoic acid and its derivatives are more effective on fair skin. For darker skin, less irritating treatment methods should be prioritized [17]. The advantage of retinoic acid derivatives is that they target both acne and hyperpigmentation [17]. The American Academy of Dermatology recommends topical retinoids for the treatment of acne and associated hyperpigmentation [17]. Retinoids inhibit tyrosinase, decrease melanin transfer, increase keratinocyte turnover, enhance stratum corneum permeability and exfoliation, break down melanin, and exhibit anti-inflammatory effects [17]. Various doses and forms of tretinoin are available, including gel at 0.01–0.1% (7 doses), cream at 0.025–0.1%, and lotion at 0.05%. There is limited research on using retinaldehyde for treating PIH related to acne; however, the 0.15% form of retinol has proven effective, while isotretinoin at 0.5% has been found to be ineffective [17]. Tazarotene is available in 0.1% gel and cream, foam, and lotion forms. Tazarotene 0.1 gel has been found to be more effective than adapalene 0.1% cream for PIH-associated acne [17]. Currently, there are no studies on the effects of trifarotene in pigmentation treatment.

The most commonly observed side effect is retinoid-associated dermatitis [11].

2.5 Bakuchiol

Bakuchiol is a 0.5% concentration of a meroterpenoid phenol purified from an Indian plant (named Babchi) seed that modulates retinoic acid receptor gene expression and collagen [18]. Additionally, it regulates the synthesis enzymes of the extracellular matrix. It also blocks the activity of α-melanocyte stimulating hormone (MSH) and tyrosinase [19].

Regarding the studies conducted with it, Bakuchiol at a 0.5% concentration used twice daily showed no difference in effectiveness for hyperpigmentation compared to a 0.5% retinol [20]. In another study, bakuchiol was found to be effective against post-inflammatory hyperpigmentation triggered by trichloroacetic acid and reduced photodamage [21].

It demonstrated similar effectiveness to retinol in antiaging spot treatments while reporting significantly fewer side effects than retinoic acid [20].

2.6 Thiamidol

Thiamidol, also known as isobutylamido thiazolyl resorcinol, is one of the strongest tyrosinase inhibitors. Additionally, it provides protection against ultraviolet B at a concentration of 0.15% [22].

In a comparative study involving 0.2% thiamidol and 4% hydroquinone, equal efficacy was found, but it was concluded that it was more effective than 2% hydroquinone [23].

0.2% thiamidol has been reported as a promising agent with good tolerance. In studies where serums and SPF 30 sunscreens containing thiamidol were used two times a day, a reduction in pigmentation was observed [24, 25].

2.7 Azelaic acid

Azelaic acid is one of the most commonly used molecules in the treatment of hyperpigmentation. Its mechanism of action involves interaction with DNA synthesis by inhibiting tyrosinase and demonstrating an anti-proliferative effect after this inhibition. It also has cytotoxic effects on abnormal melanocytes. Additionally, it exhibits anti-inflammatory properties, is against infections, and has antioxidant effects [26].

Regarding the studies conducted with azelaic acid, a 24-week multicenter controlled double-blind study involving 329 female patients showed no significant difference in efficacy between 20% azelaic acid and 4% hydroquinone with patients with melasma [27]. In another study involving 29 female patients, a comparison of 20% azelaic acid and 4% hydroquinone over a period of 2 months of treatment found azelaic acid to be more effective [27]. Also, comparing 15–20% azelaic acid with 2% hydroquinone, azelaic acid was found to be more effective, but no superiority over 4% hydroquinone was observed as the same effect was noted [27]. Additionally, another study showed that 15% azelaic acid reduces post-inflammatory hyperpigmentation caused by acne [28].

Regarding side effects, erythema was more pronounced with 4% hydroquinone at 46.6%, whereas 20% azelaic acid resulted in significantly less erythema (7.3%) [27].

2.8 Kojic acid

Kojic acid is a natural fungal metabolite used in a 1% concentration, which helps eliminate free radicals and inhibit tyrosinase. It has been found to exhibit anti-proliferative, anti-inflammatory, photoprotective, antibacterial, and antioxidant effects [29].

In studies related to spots treated with kojic acid, a controlled study on 80 patients yielded good results with 1% kojic acid and 2% hydroquinone combined with betamethasone valerate, achieving a success rate of 71.2% [30]. In another study, when examining 60 patients using either 4% hydroquinone or 0.75% kojic acid along with 2.5% ascorbic acid, better results were shown with hydroquinone after 12 weeks [31]. However, there is insufficient research to confirm kojic acid's effectiveness alone, and it is often included in combination therapies [29].

It can be recommended as an alternative for those who do not use hydroquinone.

2.9 Vitamin E

The natural forms of vitamin E consist of 4 tocopherols and 4 tocotrienols. Among these 8 isoforms, α-tocopherol is the most abundant and well-defined form found in the tissues [32]. In addition to its strong antioxidant effect, anticancer and anti-inflammatory effects have also been demonstrated [32].

Topical vitamin E is considered a potential agent that could be effective in treating hyperpigmentation. However, there is insufficient research to support its effectiveness on its own. It has predominantly been used in combination with vitamin C and other topical antioxidants, and it has been determined that these combinations could be effective in treating melasma [41].

2.10 Arbutin

Arbutin is a hydroquinone derivative found in bearberry, cranberry, and blueberry plants. Arbutin facilitates the recycling of tyrosinase activity. Forms such as α-arbutin and deoxyarbutin have been found to be effective in inhibiting tyrosinase [33].

Regarding the studies conducted with arbutin, a study involving 10 patients with melasma using 1% arbutin reported that it was effective in all treated patients [33]. Additionally, treatment with 7% α-arbutin combined with Q-switched NdYAG has also been reported as successful for melasma treatment in another study [42]. Overall, results in hyperpigmentation removal with arbutin have been found to be effective; however, the number of studies is limited.

2.11 Cysteamine

The cysteamine is an intrinsic antioxidant found in breast milk. It works by inhibiting tyrosinase and peroxidase, thereby reducing melanin formation. It is a new thiol compound that is formed by degrading L-cysteine [34, 35].

In two different randomized controlled studies conducted with cysteamine, a significant reduction in MASI was detected. In a study with 40 women with melasma, 4% hydroquinone was compared with 5% cysteamine, and hydroquinone was found to be more effective [34]. In another study comparing 4% hydroquinone with cysteamine in 20 women with melasma, more side effects were observed with cysteamine [43]. In the TCC comparison of cysteamine, equal efficacy was observed, suggesting that the cysteamine could be an alternative; more studies are needed in this era [4].

The tolerance of cysteamine is generally good. Side effects that may be observed include bad odor, erythema, dryness, pruritus, and irritation.

2.12 Glycolic acid

Glycolic acid is an alpha hydroxy acid that disrupts cell adhesion and inhibits tyrosinase. This reduces melanin production and provides desquamation [11].

In a split-face controlled study involving 21 women, the effects of a 20–30% glycolic acid peel plus 4% hydroquinone, applied every 2 weeks, were compared to 4% hydroquinone alone, with no significant difference [44]. Another study with a single-blind method with five different groups of patients showed that the combination of a 10% glycolic acid cream and 4% hydroquinone, along with 0.01% hyaluronic acid, was the most effective group; no recurrence was noted during follow-up [45].

2.13 Undecylenoyl phenylalanine

Undecylenoyl phenylalanine is a molecule formed by the combination of phenylalanine amino acid with undecylenic acid. It exerts its effects by reducing proliferation factors [11]. Additionally, it acts as an MSH antagonist by preventing MSH from binding to MCR1 receptors [11].

In studies, it has been tested as a skin tone-lightening complex along with disodium glycerophosphate, L-leucine, and phenylethyl resorcinol, resulting in a decrease in MASI scores.

Undecylenoyl phenylalanine has been reported as a well-tolerated agent for treating melasma [11].

2.14 Linoleic acid

Linoleic acid is an unsaturated omega-6 fatty acid. Linoleic acid inhibits tyrosinase, and it increases epidermal turnover at the same time [11].

In a study conducted with 47 Korean female patients using a combination cream containing linoleic acid, lincomycin, and betamethasone valerate, it was reported to reduce the melasma severity and was found to be an effective cream [11, 46].

No side effects of linoleic acid have been identified. The number of studies on the treatment of hyperpigmentation with linoleic acid is insufficient, and more research is needed [46].

2.15 Silymarin

Slymarin is obtained from the seeds of the milk thistle plant, also known as Silybum marinum, belonging to the Asteraceae family. Silymarin is a naturally occurring polyphenolic antioxidant flavonoid.

An in vitro study of a cream containing hexylresorcinol, silymarin, 20% vitamin C, and 5% vitamin E has demonstrated photoprotective effects against UVB damage [37, 47]. In another study involving silymarin, a comparative study was conducted on 42 female patients for melasma treatment using topical silymarin and hydroquinone, comparing 0.7% silymarin, 1.4% silymarin, and 4% hydroquinone cream. At the end of the 3 months, effective results were obtained in all three groups, with no significant differences reported among them [48]. While no side effects were reported with silymarin, significant side effects were noted with hydroquinone. More comprehensive studies are needed on silymarin for hyperpigmentation treatment.

2.16 Dexpanthenol

Dexpanthenol, also known as provitamin B5, can convert metabolites into energy and increase turnover in epidermal cells.

Dexpanthenol reduces spots and freckles. It was approved in 2018 as a quasi-drug for reducing melanin accumulation. However, there is currently insufficient scientific evidence for humans [29].

2.17 Glabridin

Glabridin is a natural prenylated isoflavonoid derived from *Glycyrrhiza glabra* L. (licorice). It has demonstrated anti-inflammatory, antioxidant, anti-tumor, and antimicrobial effects [49].

40 female patients with epidermal melasma applied a nonprescription priority gel formulation containing glabridin along with andrographolide and apolactoferrin twice daily for 6 months in an uncontrolled open-label study. Successful results were reported in this study [38].

No side effects were detected except for mild and temporary dryness.

2.18 Ellagic acid

Ellagic acid is a natural polyphenolic antioxidant found in certain types of fruits and tree nuts. It has demonstrated anticancer effects. Ellagic acid inhibits tyrosinase activity [29].

Ellagic acid has been used not alone but rather in combination therapies. In a randomized, prospective, open-label study conducted on 10 patients with melasma, the combination of ellagic acid and arbutin was reported to be effective in treatment [33]. While ellagic acid is a promising agent, there is insufficient research to support its effectiveness alone in the treatment of hyperpigmentation [29].

2.19 Rucinol

Rucinol (4-n-butilresorcinol) is a tyrosinase inhibitor. It also provides tyrosinase related protein (TRP) inhibition [29].

In a prospective, single-center, double-blind randomized controlled study conducted on 32 women with melasma, a significant regression was observed in the group using rucinol [50]. Additionally, a reduction in redness was also noted. 78% of the patients had a good or fair effect [50]. However, the number of studies conducted with rucinol is limited.

The tolerance of the rucinol serum is good.

2.20 Salicylic acid

Salicylic acid is an anti-inflammatory, antibacterial agent and provides non-selective inhibition of melanogenesis. Additionally, it has a protective effect against visible light and ultraviolet light. It also increases epidermal turnover. Salicylic acid is a type of beta-hydroxy acid. Due to its keratolytic effect, it is used as a peeling agent [11].

In a double-blind randomized, controlled study with 52 female patients with melasma, ellagic acid at 5% and salicylic acid at 0.1% were used with 4% hydroquinone cream twice daily for 12 weeks, and the results were compared [51]. The efficacy of 4% hydroquinone was found to be more successful in this study regarding melasma. In a single-center, investigator-blinded. In a 12-week study, a new formulation consisting of hydroxyphenoxypropionic acid, ellagic acid, yeast extract, and salicylic acid was compared with a 4% hydroquinone cream and a 0.025% tretinoin cream applied twice daily [52]. This new formulation containing salicylic acid was found to be effective, with statistically significant reductions in melasma observed in both groups.

Less redness, dryness, and peeling were reported with the new formulation.

2.21 Epidermal growth factors

Epidermal growth factors (EGF) trigger wound healing and have anti-inflammatory and antioxidant effects. It has been determined that they reduce melanin production [11].

The efficacy and safety of using an ointment containing EGFs in conjunction with a Q-switched 532 nm NdYAG laser for the treatment of solar lentigines has been evaluated [39]. In this study, patients using EGF ointment had less PIH, and its use as an adjunctive treatment after a Q-switched 532 nm laser is recommended [39]. There is not enough research demonstrating that topical products containing EGF are effective for treating spots on their own.

No significant side effects were observed for subjects using EGF ointment.

2.22 Botanical (herbal) products

Botanical (herbal) products used in the treatment of melasma have gained recognition in recent years as effective and reliable topical treatments. Some of them are already written in detail in this review.

Commonly used botanical products include polypodium, cysteamine, rucinol, glucosamine, niacinamide, soy extract, linoleic acid, licorice (glabridin), phloretin, resveratrol (mulberry and grape extracts), coffee berry, orchid, green tea leaves, eucalyptus, strawberry, silymarin, *Pinus pinaster* (pycogenol), boswellia serrata, citrus fruits (bioflavonoid, hesperidin), grape seed, aloe, sunflower seed, ginseng, Apiaceae family plants (carrot and coriander), rumex occidentalis, mulberry (Morus), and licorice (glycyrrhiza) extracts.

A meta-analysis examining botanical products in patients with melasma compiled 12 studies involving a total of 695 patients [40]. This study found significant regression in MASI scores and notable improvements in measurements using the mexameter. In this meta-analysis focused on botanical products for melasma treatment, these products were reported to be reliable and with minimal side effects. They were found to be effective for topical use. The conclusion of the study highlighted the need for more comprehensive new studies regarding the efficacy of botanical products in the treatment of melasma [40].

2.23 Trending topical ingredients combinations

In combination therapies, topical depigmenting agents most commonly include antioxidants and acids together.

A study investigating the effectiveness and tolerability of a depigmenting serum composed of tranexamic acid, niacinamide, 4-butylresorcinol, phytic acid, and hydroxyl acids found a 63% reduction in MASI scores and a 79% increase in skin luminosity [53]. This depigmenting serum has proven to be effective in the removal of the spots and is reported to have good tolerability.

Apart from phytic acid, superoxide dismutase and ferulic acid are other less commonly used antioxidants [41]. There is still insufficient research to confirm the effectiveness of these antioxidants alone for the removal of hyperpigmentation. However, these antioxidants may have a synergistic effect when combined with other antioxidants like vitamin C. A cream composed of tranexamic acid, niacinamide, ascorbyl tetraisopalmitate, glabridin, kojic acid, and arbutin, along with botanical

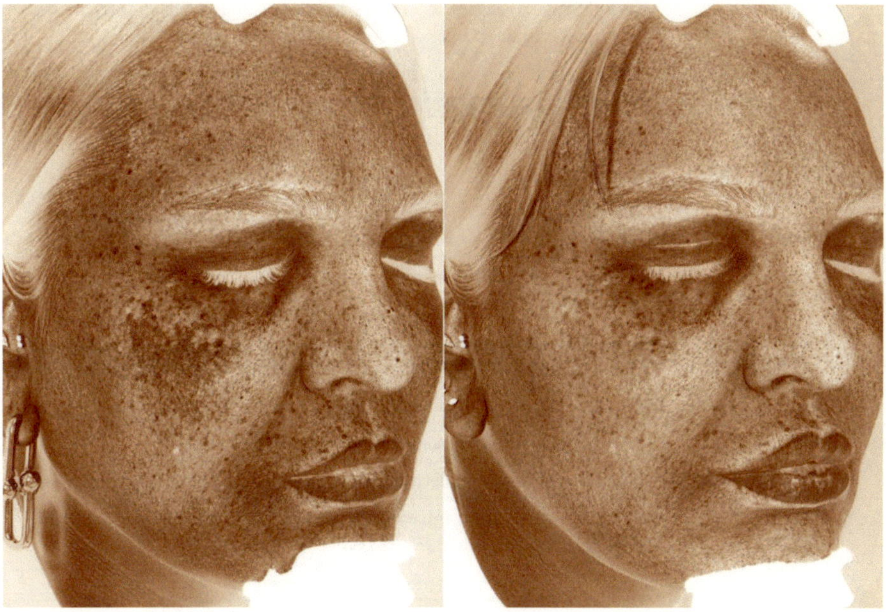

Figure 2.
Sunscreen (SPF50 + VL), ascorbic acid 2 times/day, combination cream (tranexamic acid, niacinamide, ascorbyl tetraisopalmitate, glabridin, kojic acid, arbutin, along with botanical ingredients such as Lavandula, menthe piperita, citric acid, lactobacillus, papaya fruit, and morinda citrofolia) once/day.

ingredients such as Lavandula, menthe piperita, citric acid, lactobacillus, papaya fruit, and morinda citrofolia, have also been reported as efficient in studies (**Figure 2**) [54]. There is another product that is prepared in the office for the patients' needs individually. This system allows to choose the ingredients such as niacinamide, tranexamic acid, zinc, arbutin, etc., and mix it with a serum containing 4 different types of biomimetic peptides and omega 3. Mechanisms of efficacy of trend topical ingridents are summarized in **Table 1**.

No.	Topical agent	Mechanisms of efficacy
1.	Ascorbic acid (Vitamin C)	Inhibits tyrosinase, stimulates collagen synthesis [1]
2.	Niacinamide	Prevents the transfer of melanosomes to keratinocytes, effective in reducing melanogenesis, anti-inflammatory, reduces solar degenerative changes, antiaging, emollient, protects skin barrier [8]
3.	Tranexamic acid	Reduces melanogenic factors such as prostaglandins, leukotrienes, fibroblast growth factor, α-MSH, and arachidonic acid, contributes to a reduction in CD 31+ blood vessels and endothelin, tyrosinase inhibitor, anti-inflammatory [11, 12]
4.	Retinoic acid	Inhibits tyrosinase, decreases melanin transfer, increases keratinocyte turnover, enhances stratum corneum permeability and exfoliation, breaks down melanin, and exhibits anti-inflammatory effects [17]
5.	Bakuchiol	Modulates retinoic acid receptor gene expression and collagen, regulates the synthesis enzymes of extra cellular matrix, blocks the activity of α-MSH and tyrosinase [18]
6.	Thiamidol	One of the strongest tyrosinase inhibitors, provides protection against UVB at concentration of 0.15% [25]
7.	Azelaic acid	Interaction with DNA synthesis, inhibits tyrosinase, demonstrates anti-proliferative effect, has cytotoxic effects on abnormal melanocytes, exhibits anti-inflammatory properties, is against infections, and has antioxidant effects [26]
8.	Kojic acid	Helps eliminate free radicals, inhibits tyrosinase, exhibit anti-proliferative, anti-inflammatory, photo-protective, antibacterial, antioxidant effects, UV protection [29]
9.	Vitamin E	Anti-oxidant effect, anti-cancer and anti-inflammatory effects have also been demonstrated [32]
10.	Arbutin	Facilitates the recycling of tyrosinase activity, inhibits tyrosinase [33]
11.	Cysteamine	Inhibits tyrosinase-peroxidase, reduce melanin [34, 35]
12.	Glycolic acid	Disrupts cell adhesion, inhibits tyrosinase, reduces melanin production, provides desquamation [36]
13.	Undecylenoyl phenylalanine	It exerts its effects by reducing proliferation factors. Additionally, it acts as an MSH antagonist by preventing MSH from binding to MC1R receptors [11]
14.	Linoleic acid	Inhibits tyrosinase, increases epidermal turnover at the same time [11]
15.	Silymarin	Antioxidant, photoprotective effect against UVB damage [37]
16.	Dexpanthenol	Increases turnover in epidermal cells, reduces melanin accumulation [29]
17.	Glabridin	Inhibits tyrosinase, anti-inflammatory, antioxidant, anti-tumor, calming, UV protection, anti-microbial effects [38]
18.	Ellagic acid	Demonstrated anticancer effects, inhibits tyrosinase activity [29]
19.	Rucinol	Tyrosinase inhibitor, provides TRP inhibition [29]
20.	Salisylic acid	Anti-inflammatory, provides non-selective inhibition of melanogenesis, protective effect against visible light-ultraviolet light, increases epidermal turnover, antibacterial [11]

No.	Topical agent	Mechanisms of efficacy
21.	Epidermal growth factors	Trigger wound healing, anti-inflammatory, antioxidant, reduce melanin production [39]
22.	Botanical (herbal) products	Polypodium, cisteamine, rucinol, glucosamine, niacinamide, soy extract, linoleic acid, licorice (glabridin), phloretin, resveratrol, (mulberry and grape extracts), coffee berry, orchid, green tea leaves, eucalyptus, strawberry, silymarin, pinus pinaster, (pycogenol), boswellia serrata, citrus fruits (bioflavonoid, hesperidin), grape seed, aloe, sunflower seed, ginseng, Apiaceae family plants (carrot and coriander), rumex occidentalis, mulberry (morus), licorice (glycyrrhiza) extracts are most commonly used products; they demonstare antioxidant, anti-inflammatory, photo-protective, antibacterial [40]

Table 1.
Summarizes the mechanisms of efficacy for trend topical agents for hyperpigmentation.

3. Conclusions

Today, there is a tendency to suppress melanogenesis with antioxidants and botanical products without irritating or obvious peeling of the skin. Treatments for photoaging and melasma target many steps, including UV protection, tyrosinase inhibition, inhibition of melanin transfer, anti-inflammatory effects, anti-oxidation, antiaging, increasing barrier function, protecting the skin barrier, calming, moisturizing, and collagen production. Thanks to the addition of antioxidants and antiaging products to the formulations of sunscreens developed in recent years, effective protection and treatment against hyperpigmentation can now be achieved and are easier to maintain even with a single cream.

Acknowledgements

There are no acknowledgments or funding information.

Conflict of interest

The authors declare no conflict of interest.

Abbreviations

AA	ascorbic acid
ATRA	all trans retinoic acid
EGF	epidermal growth factor
PIH	post-inflammatory hyperpigmentation
MASI	melasma area and severity index
MC1R	melanocortin 1 receptor
MSH	melanocyte stimulating hormone
TRP	tyrosinase related protein
UV	ultraviolet
VL	visible light

Author details

Özlem Karadağ Köse
Faculty of Medicine, Department of Dermatology, Istanbul Aydın University, Istanbul, Turkey

*Address all correspondence to: ozlemkkose@gmail.com

References

[1] Ko D, Wang RF, Ozog D, Lim HW, Mohammad TF. Disorders of hyperpigmentation. Part II. Review of management and treatment options for hyperpigmentation. Journal of the American Academy of Dermatology. 2023;**88**(2):291-320. DOI: 10.1016/j.jaad.2021.12.065

[2] Morgado-Carrasco D, Piquero-Casals J, Granger C, Trullas C, Passeron T. Melasma: The need for tailored photoprotection to improve clinical outcomes. Photodermatology, Photoimmunology & Photomedicine. 2022;**38**:515-521. DOI: 10.1111/phpp.12783

[3] Taylor SC, Alexis AF, Armstrong AW. Misconceptions of photoprotection in skin of color. Journal of the American Academy of Dermatology. 2022;**86**:S9-S17. DOI: 10.1016/j.jaad.2021.12.020

[4] Pennitz A, Kinberger M, Avila VG, Passeron T, Nast A, Werner RN. Self-applied topical interventions for melasma: A systematic review and meta-analysis of data from randomized, investigator-blinded clinical trials. The British Journal of Dermatology. 2022;**187**(3):309-317. DOI: 10.1111/bjd.21244

[5] Espinal-Perez LE, Moncada B, Castanedo-Cazares JP. A double-blind randomized trial of 5% ascorbic acid vs. 4% hydroquinone in melasma. International Journal of Dermatology. 2004;**43**(8):604-607. DOI: 10.1111/j.1365-4632.2004.02134.x

[6] Schwartz C, Jcan A, Zito PM. Hydroquinone. Treasure Island (FL): StatPearls Publishing LLC; 2021

[7] Hakozaki T, Minwalla L, Zhuang J, Chhoa M, Matsubora A, Greatens A, et al. The effect of niacinamide on reducing cutaneous pigmentation and supression of melanosome transfer. The British Journal of Dermatology. 2002;**147**(1):20-31. DOI: 10.1046/j.1365-2133.2002.04834.x

[8] Charoo NA. Hyperpigmentation: Looking beyond hydroquinone. Journal of Cosmetic Dermatology. 2022;**21**:4133-4145. DOI: 10.1111/jocd.14746

[9] Navarrete-Solis J, Castanedo-Cazares JP, Torres-Alvarez B, Oros-Ovalle C, Fuentes-Ahumada C, Gonzalez FJ, et al. A double-blind, randomized clinical tral of niacinamide 4% versus hydroquinone 4% in the treatment of melasma. Dermatology Research and Practice. 2011;**21**:379173. DOI: 10.1155/2011/379173

[10] Campuzano-Garcia AE, Torres-Alvarez B, Hernandez-Blanco D, Fuentes-Ahumada C, Cortes-Garcia JD, Castanedo-Cazares JP. DNA methyltransferases in malar melasma and their modification by sunscreen in combination with 4% niacinamide, 0.05% retinoic acid, or placebo. BioMed Research International. 2019:9068314. DOI: 10.1155/2019/9068314

[11] Gonzalez-Molina V, Marti-Pineda A, Noelina G. Topical treatment for melasma and their mechanism of action. The Journal of Clinical And Aesthetic Dermatology. 2022;**15**(5):19-28

[12] Kanechorn Na AP, Niumphradit N, Manosroi A, Nakakes A. Topical 5% tranexamic acid for the treatment of melasma in Asians: A double-blind randomized controlled clinical trial. Journal of Cosmetic and Laser Therapy. 2012;**14**(3):150-154. DOI: 10.3109/14764172.2012.685478

[13] Lindgren AL, Austin AH, Welsh KM. The use of tranexamic acid to prevent and treat post-inflammatory hyperpigmentation. Journal of Drugs in Dermatology. 2021;**20**(3):344-345. DOI: 10.36849/JDD.5622

[14] Ebrahimi B, Naeini FF. Topical tranexamic acid as a promising treatment for melasma. Journal of Research in Medical Sciences: The Official Journal of Isfahan University of Medical Sciences. 2014;**19**(8):753-757

[15] Atefi N, Dalvant B, Ghassemi M, Mehran G, Heydarian A. Therapeutic effects of topical tranexamic acid in comparison with hydroquinone in treatment of women with melasma. Dermatologic Therapy. 2017;**7**(3):417-424. DOI: 10.1007/s13555-017-0195-0

[16] Banihashemi M, Zabolinejad N, Jaafari MR, Salehi M, Jabari A. Comparison of therapeutic effects of liposomal tranexamic acid and conventional hydroquinone on melasma. Journal of Cosmetic Dermatology. 2015;**14**(3):174-177. DOI: 10.1111/jocd.12152

[17] Callender VD, Baldwin H, Cook-Bolden FE, Alexis AF, Stein GL, Guenin E. Effects of topical retinoids on acne and post-inflammatory hyperpigmentation in patients with skin of color: A clinical review and implications for practice. American Journal of Clinical Dermatology. 2022;**23**(1):69-81. DOI: 10.1007/s40257-021-00643-2

[18] Chaudhuri RK, Bojanowski K. Bakuchiol: A retinol-like functional compound revealed by gene expression profilling and clinically proven to have anti-aging effects. International Journal of Cosmetic Science. 2014;**36**(3):221-230. DOI: 10.1111/ics.12117

[19] Ohno O, Watabe T, Nakamura K, Kawagoshi M, et al. Inhibitory effects of bakuchiol, bavachin, and isobavachalcone isolated from *Piper longum* on melanin production in B16 mouse melanoma cells. Bioscience, Biotechnology, and Biochemistry. 2010;**74**(7):1504-1506. DOI: 10.1271/bbb.100221

[20] Dhaliwal S, Rybak I, Ellis SR, Notay M, Trivedi M, Burney W, et al. Prospective, randomized, double-blind assessment of topical bakuchiol and retinol for facial photoageing. The British Journal of Dermatology. 2019;**180**(2):289-296. DOI: 10.1111/bjd.16918

[21] Lyons AB, Kohli I, Nahhas AF, Braunberger TL, Mohammad TF, Nicholson CL, et al. Trichloroacetic acid model to accurately capture the efficacy of treatments for postinflammatory hyperpigmentation. Archives of Dermatological Research. 2020;**312**(10):725-730. DOI: 10.1007/s00403-020-02071-4

[22] Vachiramon V, Sakpuwadol N, Yongpisarn T, Anuntrangsee T, Palakornkitti P. Efficacy of isobutylamido thiazolyl resorcinol for prevention of laser-induced post-inflammatory hyperpigmentation: A randomized, controlled trial. Journal of Cosmetic Dermatology. 2024;**23**(7):2450-2457. DOI: 10.1111/jocd.16287

[23] Lima PB, Dias JAF, Cassiano DP, Esposito ACC, Miot LDB, Bagatin E, et al. Efficacy and safety of topical isobutylamido thiazolyl resorcinol (Thiamidol) vs. 4% hydroquinone cream for facial melasma: An evaluator-blinded, randomized controlled trial. Journal of the European Academy of Dermatology and Venereology. 2021;**35**(9):1881-1887. DOI: 10.1111/jdv.17344

[24] Arrowitz C, Schoelermann AM, Mann T, Jiang LI, Weber T, Kolbe L.

Effective tyrosinase inhibition by yhiamidol results in significant improvement of mild to moderate melasma. The Journal of Investigative Dermatology. 2019;**139**(8):1691-1698. DOI: 10.1016/j.jid.2019.02.013

[25] Vachiramon V, Kositkuljorn C, Leerunyakul CK. Isobutylamido thiazolyl resorcinol for prevention of UVB-induced hyperpigmentation. Journal of Cosmetic Dermatology. 2021;**20**(3):987-992. DOI: 10.1111/jocd.13615

[26] Gupta AK, Gover MD, Nouri K, Taylor S. The treatment of melasma: A review of clinical trials. Journal of the American Academy of Dermatology. 2006;**55**(6):1048-1065. DOI: 10.1016/j.jaad.2006.02.009

[27] Balina LM, Graupe K. The treatment of melasma. 20% azeleic acid versus 4% hydroquinone cream. International Journal of Dermatology. 1991;**30**(12):893-895. DOI: 10.1111/j.1365-4362.1991.tb04362.x

[28] Kircik LH. Efficacy and safety of azelaic acid (AzA) gel 15% in the treatment of post-inflammatory hyperpigmentation and acne: A 16-week, baseline-controlled study. Journal of Drugs in Dermatology. 2011;**10**(6):586-590

[29] Maeda K. Timeline of the development of skin lightening active ingridednts in Japan. Molecules. 2022;**27**:4774. DOI: 10.3390/molecules27154774

[30] Saeedi M, Eslamifar M, Khezri K. Kojic acid applications in cosmetic and pharmaceutical preperations. Biomedicine & Pharmacotherapy. 2019;**110**:582-593. DOI: 10.1016/j.biopha.2018.12.006

[31] Monteiro RC, Kishore BN, Bhat RM, Sukumar D, Martis J, Ganesh HK. A comparative study of the efficacy of 4% hydroquinone vs 0.75% Kojic acid cream in the treatment of facial melasma. Indian Journal of Dermatology. 2013;**58**(2):157. DOI: 10.4103/0019-5154.108070

[32] Jang Y, Kim CY. The role of vitamin E isoforms and metabolites in cancer prevention: Mechanistic insights into syphingolipid metabolism modulation. Nutrients. 2024;**16**(23):4115. DOI: 10.3390/nu16234115

[33] Ertam SI, Mutlu B, Unal I, Alper S, Kıvçak B, Özer Ö. Efficiency of ellagic acid and arbutin in melasma: A randomized, prospective, open label study. Journal of Dermatology. 2008;**35**:570-574. DOI: 10.1111/j.1346-8138.2008.00522.x

[34] Lima PB, Dias JAF, Cassiano D, Esposito ACC, Bagatin E, Miot LDB, et al. A comparative study of topical 5% cysteamine versus 4% hydroquinone in the treatment of facial melasma in women. International Journal of Dermatology. 2020;**59**(12):1531-1536. DOI: 10.1111/ijd.15146

[35] Gan C, Rodrigues M. An update on new and existing treatments for the management of melasma. American Journal of Clinical Dermatology. 2024;**25**:717-733. DOI: 10.1007/s40257-024-00863-2

[36] Cassiano DP, ACC E, da Silva C, Lima PM, JAF D, Hassun K, et al. Update on melasma-part II: treatment. Dermatology Treatment (Heidelb). 2022;**12**(9):1989-2012. DOI: 10.1007/s13555-022-00780-4

[37] Draelos ZD, Diaz I, Cohen A, Mao J, Boyd T. A novel skin brightening topical technology. Journal of Cosmetic Dermatology. 2020;**19**(12):3280-3285. DOI: 10.1111/jocd.13741

[38] Cantelli M, Ferrillo M, Donnarumma M, Emanuele E, Fabbrocini G. A new proprietary gel containing glabridin, andrographolide, and apolactoferrin improves the appearance of epidermal melasma in adult women: A 6-month pilot, uncontrolled open-labelled study. Journal of Cosmetic Dermatology. 2023;**19**(6):1395-1398. DOI: 10.1111/jocd.13161

[39] Kim HO, Kim HR, Kim JC, Kang SY, Jung MJ, Chang SE, et al. A randomized controlled trial on the effectiveness of epidermal growth factor containing oinment on the treatment of solar lentigines as adjuvant therapy. Medicina (Kaunas, Lithuania). 2021;**57**(166):1-11

[40] Furmanczyk M, Brown A, Bustos J, Fernandes de Henestosa AR, Trullas C, Granger C, et al. Efficacy and tolerability of a depigmanting gel serum comprising tranexamic acid, niacinamide, 4-butylresorcinol, phytic acid, and a mixture of hydroxy acids that targets the biological processes regulating skin melanogenesis. Journal of Cosmetic Dermatology. 2024;**23**:2058-2065. DOI: 10.1111/jocd.16148

[41] Babbush KM, Babbush RA, Khachemoune A. Treatment of melasma: A review of less commonly used antioxidants. International Journal of Dermatology. 2021;**60**(2):166-173. DOI: 10.1111/ijd.15133

[42] Polnikorn N. Treatment of refractory melasma with the MedLite C6 Q-switched Nd:YAG laser and alpha arbutin: A prospective study. Journal of Cosmetic and Laser Therapy. 2010;**12**(3):126-131. DOI: 10.3109/14764172.2010.487910

[43] Nguyen J, Remyn L, Chung IY, Honigman A, Gourani-Tehrani S, Wutami I, et al. Evaluation of the efficacy of cysteamine cream compared to hydroquinone in the treatment of melasma: A randomised, double-blinded trial. The Australasian Journal of Dermatology. 2021;**62**(1):e41-e46. DOI: 10.1111/ajd.13432

[44] Hurley ME, Guevara IL, Gonzalez RM, et al. Efficacy of glycolic acid peels in the treatment of melasma. Archives of Dermatology. 2002;**138**(12):1578-1582. DOI: 10.1001/archderm.138.12.1578

[45] Ibrahim ZA, Gheida SF, El Maghraby GM, Farag ZE. Evaluation of the efficacy and safety of combinations of hydroquinone, glycolic acid, and hyaluronic acid in the treatment of melasma. Journal of Cosmetic Dermatology. 2015;**14**(2):113-123. DOI: 10.1111/jocd.12143

[46] Lee MH, Kim HJ, Ha DJ, Paik JH, Kim HY. Therapeutic effect of topical application of linoleic acid and lincomycin in combination with betamethasone valerate in melasma patients. Journal of Korean Medical Science. 2002;**17**(4):518-523. DOI: 10.3346/jkms.2002.17.4.518

[47] Draelos ZD, Kerscher M, Lynch S, White S, Choudhary H. A Silymarin antioxidant serum improves facial acne alone and as part of a treatment regimen. Journal of Drugs in Dermatology. 2024;**23**(4):233-238. DOI: 10.36849/JDD.8120

[48] Nofal A, Ibrahim AM, Nofal E, Gamal N, Osman S. Topical silymarin versus hydroquinone in the treatment of melasma: A comparative study. Journal of Cosmetic Dermatology. 2019;**18**(1):263-270. DOI: 10.1111/jocd.12769

[49] Zhang J, Wu X, Zhong B, Liao Q, Wang X, Xie Y, et al. Review on the diverse biological effects of glabridin.

Drug Design, Development and Therapy. 2023;**10**:15-37. DOI: 10.2147/DDDT.S385981

[50] Khemis A, Kaiafa A, Queille-Roussel C, Duteil L, Ortonne JP. Evaluation of efficacy and safety of rucinol serum in patients with melasma: A randomized controlled trial. The British Journal of Dermatology. 2007;**156**(5):997-1004. DOI: 10.1111/j.1365-2133.2007.07814.x

[51] Dahl A, Yatskayer M, Raab S, Oresajo C. Tolerance and efficacy of a product containing ellagic and salicylic acids in reducing hyperpigmentation and dark spots in comparison with 4% hydroquinone. Journal of Drugs in Dermatology. 2013;**12**(1):52-58

[52] Draelos Z, Dahl A, Yatskayer M. Dyspigmentation, skin physiology and a movel approach to skin lightening. Journal of Cosmetic Dermatology. 2013;**12**(4):247-253. DOI: 10.1111/jocd.12066

[53] Wang T, Wang Y, Wang J, Chen H, Qu B, Li Z. Efficacy and safety of topical therapy with botanical products for melasma: A systematic review and meta-analysis of randomized controlled trials. Frontiers in Medicine. 2022;**8**:1-11. DOI: 10.3389/fmed.2021.797890

[54] Shariff R, Du Y, Dutta M, Kumar S, Thimmaiah S, Doraiswamy C, et al. Superior even skin tone and anti-ageing benefit of a combination of 4-hexylresorcinol and niacnamide. International Journal of Cosmetic Science. 2022;**44**(1):103-117. DOI: 10.1111/ics.12759

Chapter 9

Lip Filler: Anatomy, Techniques, and Management of Complications

Francesco Castellaneta and Mariagiovanna Lombardi

Abstract

Hyaluronic acid-based lip fillers are one of the most sought-after minimally invasive esthetic treatments to enhance lip volume, contour, and hydration. This chapter examines lip anatomy, aging processes, and key injection techniques, providing a comprehensive overview of the safest and most effective methodologies. Different injection techniques are illustrated, including the linear retrograde method, the microbolus technique, and the cannula approach, highlighting their advantages and potential risks. Special attention is given to complications, ranging from minor inflammatory reactions to vascular occlusions, analyzing prevention strategies and emergency management protocols, such as the use of hyaluronidase to dissolve the filler in case of adverse events. Finally, the chapter emphasizes the importance of proper practitioner training and thorough patient assessment to achieve natural and safe results. The continuous evolution of techniques and materials is increasingly improving the quality and longevity of outcomes, making the treatment a safe and effective option when performed by qualified professionals.

Keywords: filler, hyaluronic acid (HA), lip rejuvenation, skin rejuvenation, filler lips

1. Introduction

In recent decades, the use of lip fillers has become increasingly popular in the field of esthetic medicine, representing one of the most requested minimally invasive procedures. The desire for fuller, more defined, and harmonious lips is driven not only by evolving esthetic standards but also by the influence of social media and celebrities.

Hyaluronic acid (HA)-based fillers are now considered the gold standard choice for lip treatment due to their safety, reversibility, and ability to deliver natural results [1]. However, the lip filler procedure is not limited to simple volume enhancement; it involves a range of refined techniques to improve the shape, symmetry, and projection of the lips based on the individual characteristics of the patient.

2. Anatomy

The esthetic appearance of the lips is determined by several morphological features:

- *Vermilion*: The red and visible portion of the lips, lacking sebaceous and sweat glands.
- *Vermilion-cutaneous border*: The transition between the skin and vermilion, a prominent line that defines the lip contour.
- *Cupid's bow*: The double curve on the upper lip, defined by the columns of the filter.
- *Columns of the filter*: Two vertical skin ridges that run from the upper lip to the base of the nose.
- *Labial commissures*: The lateral points of connection between the upper and lower lips.

The lips consist of multiple overlapping layers, including:

- *Epidermis*: Thin and rich in nerve endings, with high tactile sensitivity.
- *Dermis*: Contains fibroblasts, collagen, and elastin, which are essential for skin tone.
- *Subcutaneous tissue*: Includes a thin layer of fat, more prominent in the lower lip.

The most important muscle of the lips is the *orbicularis oris*, which surrounds the oral opening and allows for lip closure, protrusion, and compression.

In addition to the orbicularis oris, several muscular structures contribute to lip movements:

- *Levator labii superioris*: Lifts the upper lip.
- *Zygomaticus major and minor*: Involved in smiling.
- *Buccinator*: Contributes to lip mobility and chewing function.
- *Depressor labii inferioris*: Lowers the lower lip.

The vascularization of the lips is provided by branches of the facial artery, namely:

- *Superior labial artery*: Follows the border of the upper lip.
- *Inferior labial artery*: Runs along the lower lip.
- *Anastomosis between labial arteries*: Ensures a wide network of blood supply.

These arteries run primarily between the orbicularis oris muscle and the labial mucosa (80%), with potential anatomical variations that must be considered to avoid complications in esthetic procedures such as filler injections [2–5].

The sensory innervation of the lips is provided by branches of the *trigeminal nerve (V cranial nerve)*:

- *Infraorbital nerve* (branch of the maxillary nerve, V2): Innervates the upper lip.
- *Mental nerve* (branch of the mandibular nerve, V3): Innervates the lower lip.

Motor innervation is provided by the *facial nerve (VII cranial nerve)*, responsible for controlling the mimetic muscles.

2.1 Implications in esthetic surgery

To avoid vascular complications, it is advisable to inject the filler superficially, at a depth of less than 3 mm. Medially, the labial artery is more superficial, increasing the risk of accidental intravascular injection. It is preferable to use the *linear threading technique* along the cutaneous-vermilion border.

2.2 Lip lifting

Lip lift procedures must preserve the integrity of the *orbicularis oris muscle* to prevent visible scarring. Preoperative planning should consider the position of the *labial arteries* to minimize bleeding.

2.3 Correction of perioral wrinkles

Smoker's lines can be treated with low-G' fillers to achieve a natural effect. Botulinum toxin can be used to relax the *orbicularis oris muscle* and prevent excessive contractions.

3. Preliminary evaluation

Before performing any filler treatment, it is essential to carry out a detailed assessment of the patient. This includes a *structural analysis*, which involves evaluating the occlusal plane and its influence on the position of the lips, identifying any lip asymmetries that could affect the final result, and considering the dental arrangement, including any edentulous areas or prostheses that may alter lip support.

In addition, a thorough *pharmacological and medical history* must be taken. Special attention should be given to patients on *Oral Anticoagulant Therapy (OAT)*, as this poses a risk for bruising and hematomas. It is also important to consider any *autoimmune diseases* (such as Scleroderma), as these conditions can lead to reduced skin elasticity and compromised vascularization, which may impact the procedure's outcome.

3.1 Lip aging and structural changes

Lip aging is a complex physiological process involving a series of structural modifications at the cutaneous, mucosal, and osseous levels. Over time, the lips undergo a progressive loss of volume, definition, and firmness due to both intrinsic (genetic and biological) and extrinsic (environmental and lifestyle-related) factors. These changes not only affect the labial mucosa but also the perioral area, leading to the appearance of wrinkles, reduced elasticity, and the loss of structural support.

Understanding the processes underlying lip aging is essential for planning targeted and personalized treatments, such as hyaluronic acid-based fillers, which can restore volume and definition in a harmonious and natural way.

3.1.1 Intrinsic and extrinsic aging processes

Lip aging is determined by two main categories of factors:

- *Intrinsic aging*: This is the natural and biological process regulated by genetics and physiological changes that occur over time. It includes the reduction in collagen and elastin production, bone resorption, and changes in adipose tissue composition.
- *Extrinsic aging*: This is related to environmental factors and lifestyle habits that accelerate the aging process. The most relevant contributors include UV exposure, smoking, pollution, diet, and repetitive muscle movements that promote the formation of static and dynamic wrinkles.

These two mechanisms interact, progressively altering the anatomical and functional characteristics of the lips.

3.1.2 Loss of collagen and elastin

Collagen and elastin are two essential proteins for maintaining tissue structure and elasticity. With aging:

- *Type I and III collagen*, the primary components of the extracellular matrix, progressively decrease, leading to a loss of firmness and volume.
- *Elastin*, responsible for the skin's ability to retract after stretching, degrades, contributing to the formation of wrinkles and sagging of the lip contour.

Studies show that from the age of 25, collagen production declines by approximately 1% per year, with a significant acceleration after menopause in women. The reduction of these proteins results in a progressive loss of structural support in the lips, making them appear less full and more prone to wrinkle formation.

3.1.3 Thinning of the labial mucosa

The labial mucosa, unlike the surrounding skin, is thinner and lacks a well-developed stratum corneum, making it particularly vulnerable to the effects of aging. Over time, the following changes occur: a reduction in mucosal thickness, leading to a loss of volume and hydration; alterations in endogenous hyaluronic acid production, reducing the ability to retain water and decreasing lip turgor; and decreased vascularization, giving the lips a less rosy and more dull appearance.

These changes make the lips more prone to dryness, flaking, and loss of contour definition.

3.1.4 Bone resorption and structural support modifications

A frequently overlooked aspect of lip aging is the change occurring in the facial skeleton. Bone resorption affects the shape and projection of the lips, particularly at the maxilla and mandible levels. The *alveolar process of the maxilla* undergoes progressive resorption, reducing support for the upper lip. Bone retraction contributes to the loss of upper lip projection, making it appear less prominent and flatter. The chin tends to shrink and retract, causing a less defined jawline and a tendency for the lower face to collapse. The loss of bone support accentuates the formation of wrinkles in the perioral area and the appearance of deeper nasolabial folds.

These bone changes, combined with the loss of subcutaneous fat tissue, lead to a global alteration in lip and perioral structure.

3.2 Effects of aging on the lips and perioral area

The described structural modifications result in a series of visible changes that affect the appearance of the lips and surrounding areas.

One of the most noticeable effects of aging is the gradual and progressive loss of lip volume. This phenomenon is due to a combination of:

- Decreased subcutaneous adipose tissue.
- Reduced synthesis of hyaluronic acid, collagen, and elastin.
- Loss of bone support.

The lips become thinner, less prominent, and less defined in appearance.

The vertical wrinkles that form on the upper lip, known as *"barcode wrinkles,"* are one of the most characteristic manifestations of perioral aging. Their onset is due to:

- *Repeated muscle movements*, particularly in individuals with strong activity of the orbicularis oris muscle.
- *Loss of elastin and collagen*, reducing the skin's ability to return to its original position after muscle contraction.
- *Decreased structural support*, making the skin more prone to sagging and static wrinkle formation.

Factors such as smoking and sun exposure accelerate the appearance of these wrinkles, making them deeper and more visible.

The *vermilion*, or the visible part of the labial mucosa, undergoes significant changes with age:

- *Eversion of the upper lip decreases*, leading to a flatter and less prominent appearance.
- *The transition between skin and mucosa becomes less defined*, resulting in the loss of lip contour.
- *The Cupid's bow appears less pronounced*, altering the harmony of the upper lip.

These changes contribute to an aged and less youthful facial appearance.

4. Product selection and treatment protocol

The most commonly used filler for lips is hyaluronic acid, which ensures safety, reversibility, and a natural effect. The choice of product density varies according to specific goals: low- or medium-G' fillers are ideal for hydration and treating superficial wrinkles, while medium- or high-G' fillers are better suited for contouring and volumizing. A personalized protocol is essential for achieving harmonious results, always considering the natural dynamics of the lips and the individual needs of each patient [6–8].

The choice of injection technique is crucial for achieving optimal results. Various methods exist, each with specific indications:

- *Linear technique (Retrotracing)*: The needle is inserted parallel to the lip, and the filler is injected gradually while withdrawing the syringe. This technique is ideal for redefining the lip contour and achieving uniform filling.

- *Vertical technique (Paris Lips)*: Injections are performed perpendicular to the lip, creating vertical support columns for a more natural and structured effect. This technique is useful for correcting a thinning upper lip.

- *Serial technique*: This involves injecting the filler through multiple small punctures, one after the other, to achieve a distributed and natural filling.

- *Russian lips technique*: Characterized by microinjections placed vertically along the vermilion border, with a special emphasis on the upper lip and Cupid's bow. The result is high, flat, well-defined lips without excessive forward projection.

The choice of injection technique for lip augmentation depends on various factors, including the desired outcome, the patient's lip anatomy, and the expertise of the practitioner. Several approaches can be used, each offering unique benefits and considerations.

One of the most common and versatile techniques is the *linear retrograde injection*, where the needle is inserted into the tissue, and filler is deposited while slowly withdrawing. This method ensures even distribution of the product along the injection path, making it ideal for defining the vermilion border, enhancing contours, and achieving subtle volume augmentation. However, it requires precision to avoid overcorrection and, if performed too superficially, may lead to increased bruising.

For broader volume distribution, the *fan technique (fanning)* is often preferred. This approach involves multiple linear retrograde injections originating from a single entry point, allowing the filler to spread evenly in different directions. Frequently used in the lower lip, it creates a uniform plump effect while reducing trauma and bruising due to fewer injection sites. However, achieving balanced results requires an experienced injector, as improper execution can lead to uneven distribution.

In cases where a more natural integration of the filler is desired, the *microbolus (microdroplet) technique* is an effective option. By injecting small amounts of filler in multiple tiny deposits across the lips, this method enhances hydration and smoothness rather than adding dramatic volume. While it minimizes the risk of visible lumps and overcorrection, it involves more injection points, which may lead to increased bruising and is not suitable for patients seeking a significant volumizing effect.

A highly specialized approach that has gained popularity is the *Russian Lips technique*, designed to create a lifted, heart-shaped lip appearance without excessive forward projection. Unlike traditional horizontal injections, this method involves placing microdroplets of filler vertically along the vermilion to enhance lip height rather than bulk. While the results are highly defined and reduce the risk of migration, the technique is more complex and time-consuming, with an increased likelihood of swelling due to multiple injections.

For patients primarily seeking improved lip hydration rather than a change in shape or volume, the *hydration technique (skinbooster for lips)* is a suitable choice. Using low-viscosity, non-crosslinked, or lightly crosslinked hyaluronic acid fillers, this method involves superficial microinjections that enhance moisture retention and improve lip softness and smoothness [9]. While the risk of overcorrection is minimal, the results are subtle and may require multiple sessions to achieve the desired effect.

By carefully selecting the appropriate injection approach based on individual patient needs, practitioners can achieve esthetically pleasing results while minimizing potential complications. Each technique offers distinct advantages, and mastering their application ensures optimal lip enhancement tailored to each patient's unique facial structure and esthetic goals.

When injecting the upper lip, it is essential to consider the depth of the artery rather than its exact anatomical position. The superficial labial artery runs between the orbicularis muscle and the labial mucosa, or sometimes within the muscle itself. A linear injection technique is recommended, at or slightly below the cutaneous-vermilion border, with a depth of less than 3 mm. A soft filler with intermediate or low G' is preferable, as it distributes easily, reducing the risk of irregularities.

This technique allows for volume enhancement and improved definition of the cutaneous-vermilion border. In cases of volume deficiency, the needle can be directed deeper into the dry vermilion or injected directly at that level while maintaining a superficial and linear technique. Laterally, the artery usually runs above the vermilion border, but as it passes through Cupid's bow, it can be located between 1 and 4 mm below the vermilion border [10].

Medially, superficial injection is crucial, as the needle is much closer to the artery compared to the lateral zone. Additionally, in this area, small septal branches from the superficial labial artery may pass over the orbicularis muscle.

Fine wrinkles on the upper lip, known as "smoker's lines," can be treated with a low-G' filler, injected at the dermal level starting from the cutaneous-vermilion border using the linear threading technique. The same principles apply to the lower lip. Superficial injections should not exceed a depth of 3 mm in the cutaneous-vermilion junction area, using a low- or intermediate-G' filler and the linear threading technique [10].

To achieve the best results, many patients benefit from treatment across multiple anatomical subunits, avoiding the "quilted" effect that occurs when only one isolated area is treated. With our "U-technique," we inject the labial commissure at the superficial subcutaneous level, continuing into the lateral third of the upper and lower lips.

4.1 When to choose a needle vs. a cannula

The choice between a *needle* and a *cannula* for lip filler injections depends on the specific technique and the desired outcome.

- *For defining the vermilion border*, a *needle* is the preferred option because of its precision in placing filler along the lip contours. Cannulas are less effective in this area due to their blunt tip, which makes it harder to achieve sharp definition.

- *For volume augmentation*, both *needles and cannulas* can be used effectively. Needles provide precise placement, while cannulas offer a more uniform distribution of filler with fewer injection points, reducing trauma.

- *For hydration treatments (skinboosters)*, both *needles and cannulas* are viable choices, depending on the depth and technique used.

- *For the Russian lips technique*, which involves vertical injections to lift the lips rather than simply adding volume, a *needle* is required. Cannulas are not suitable for this method.

- *For minimizing trauma and bruising*, a *cannula* is the better option, as its blunt tip reduces the risk of vascular injury and requires fewer entry points.

Many practitioners choose to combine both techniques, using needles for contouring and definition and cannulas for volume augmentation and improved safety. This hybrid approach allows for precise shaping while minimizing trauma and the risk of complications.

4.2 "4.3 technique"

This methodology is suitable for a wide range of patients, both men and women, with standard anatomical characteristics who wish to enhance the contour of the upper and lower lip in the pale/vermilion zones [11]. The goal is to achieve a more precise definition of the Cupid's bow and philtral columns, ensuring a more harmonious projection and increasing lip volume while maintaining a smooth, elegant effect without excessive fullness.

Lip shape and volume are optimized through needle injections that gently lift the so-called "White Lip Roll," the lighter and softer tissue located just above the vermilion. This approach enhances the contour in the canine region without creating a "duck beak" effect. Additionally, the philtrum profile can be refined by adjusting the curvature of the lip without the need for direct injections into the philtral columns.

The technique involves a combination of retrograde linear and vertical needle injections at specific points: four in the upper lip and three in the lower lip. The treatment employs a hyaluronic acid-based filler (Art Filler Lips® with 0.3% lidocaine), which, thanks to Tri-Hyal technology, allows for the desired outcome to be achieved.

The first injection is administered at the peak of the right Cupid's bow, directed medially toward the superior labial tubercle. Using the retrograde linear technique, a controlled amount of hyaluronic acid is injected to volumize the muscular plane of the lip, forming a columnar structure that helps evert and enhance the upper lip. From the same entry point, the needle is then inserted laterally along the vermilion border in a subcutaneous plane, releasing the filler using the same technique to improve contour definition. The lateral portion is treated through an additional entry point, again using the retrograde linear technique. The same procedure is mirrored on the opposite side of the upper lip to ensure symmetry (**Figure 1**).

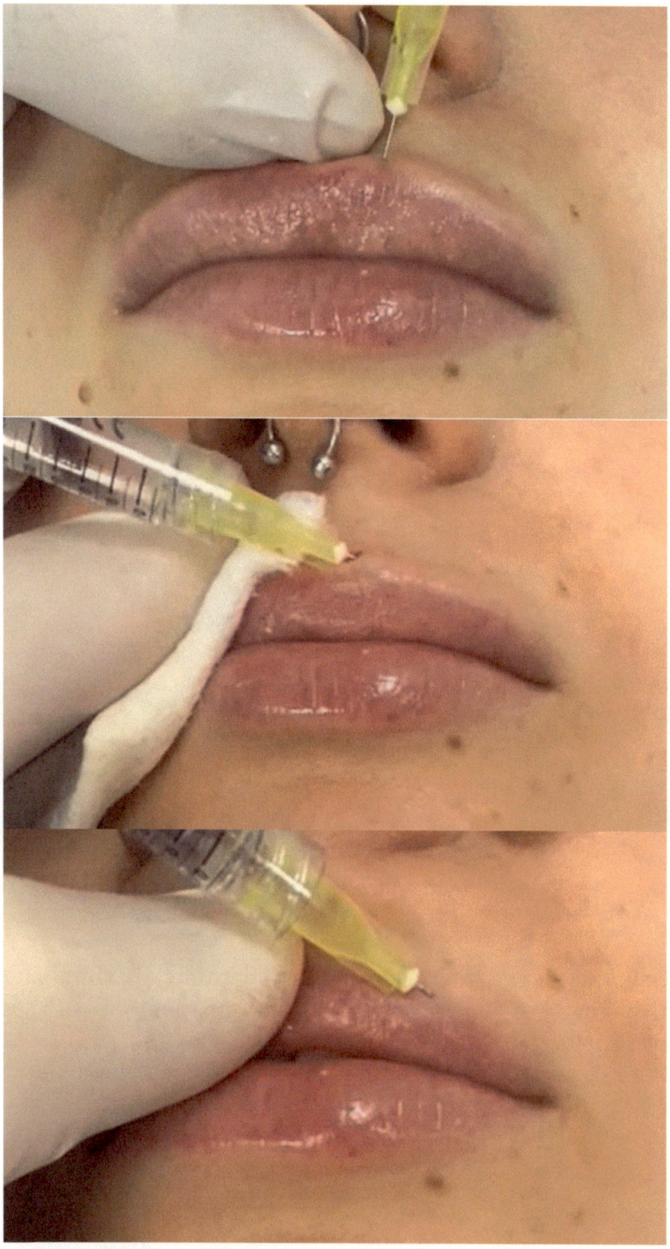

Figure 1.
Injection sequence for the upper lip.

For the lower lip, three injections are performed: one at the center of the vermilion border and the other two at intermediate positions between the two hemilips, also along the vermilion margin (**Figure 2**). The combined technique, which integrates vertical and retrograde linear injections, ensures an even distribution of the filler. It is essential to carefully control the injection depth to avoid superficial irregularities or vascular complications associated with overly deep infiltration.

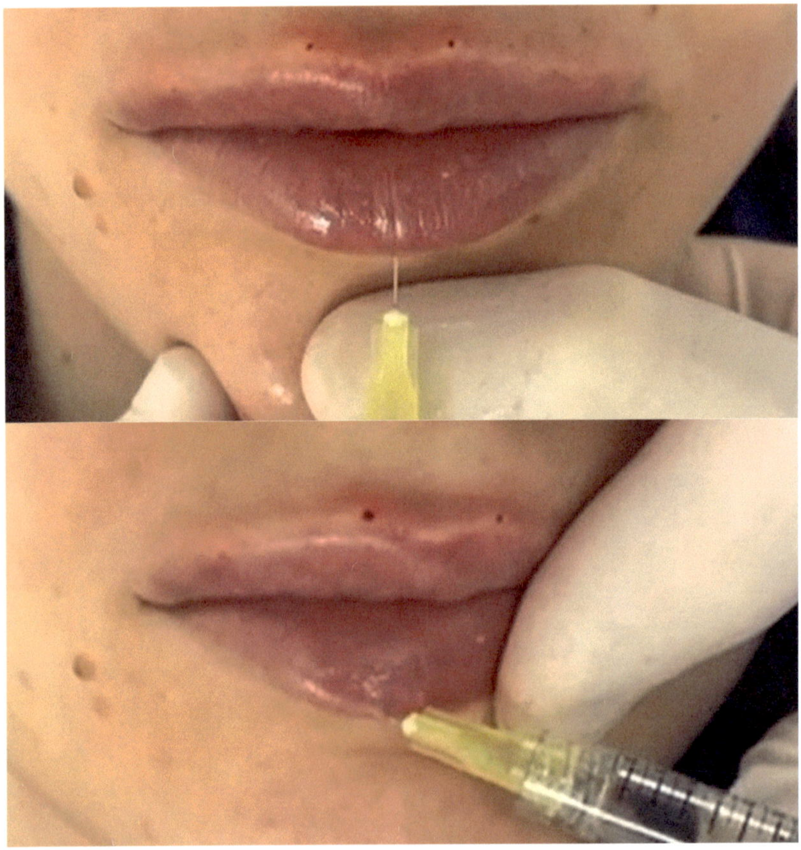

Figure 2.
Injection sequence for the lower lip.

The "4.3 technique" is characterized by its standardization, simplicity, and intuitive approach, making it easily reproducible for most patients of both sexes. This method achieves a natural appearance with a minimal amount of filler (approximately 0.7 ml) and a limited number of injection points, ensuring a less invasive treatment for the patient (**Figures 3** and **4**).

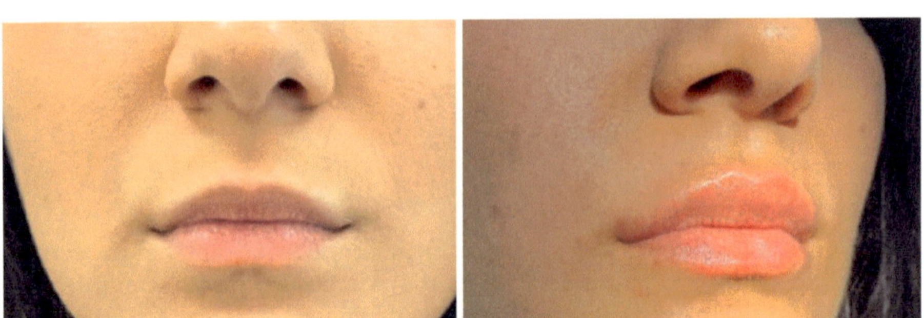

(a) (b)

Figure 3.
Case: 1 (a) Before Treatment; and (b) Follow-up 3 months after the treatment.

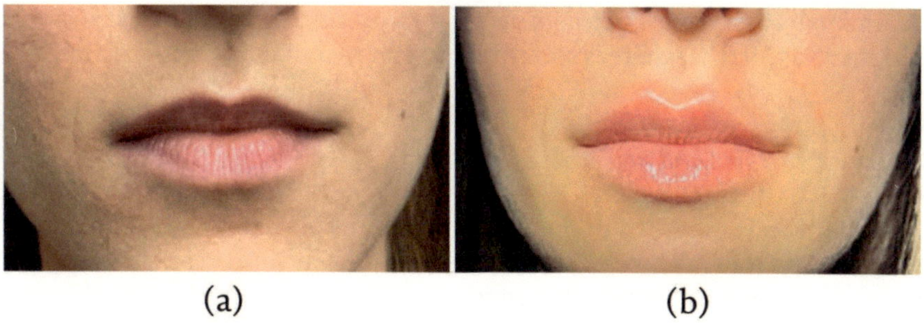

Figure 4.
Case: 2 (a) Before Treatment; and (b) Follow-up 3 months after the treatment.

5. Complications of lip fillers

5.1 Management of complications in lip filler injections

Lip filler procedures, when performed by trained professionals, are generally safe and well-tolerated. However, as with any cosmetic or medical intervention, complications can occur. These complications range from minor and self-limiting issues, such as swelling and bruising, to more serious concerns like vascular occlusion and granuloma formation. Proper management of these complications is crucial for ensuring patient safety, optimizing esthetic outcomes, and maintaining confidence in non-surgical cosmetic procedures.

A proactive approach is key to minimizing risks and addressing complications effectively when they arise. Prevention through safe injection techniques and knowledge of vascular anatomy plays a crucial role in avoiding serious complications. However, if an issue does occur, early recognition and intervention can significantly reduce the severity of adverse outcomes. This chapter explores the strategies for preventing complications, managing minor side effects, addressing vascular emergencies, and treating delayed reactions such as nodules and granulomas.

5.2 Preventive strategies

The best way to manage complications is to prevent them from occurring in the first place. Safe injection techniques, an understanding of high-risk areas, and appropriate product selection all contribute to reducing the likelihood of complications.

5.2.1 Safe injection techniques

One of the most effective ways to minimize risk is by adopting proper injection techniques. Injecting slowly is essential, as rapid injections increase the likelihood of vascular compromise and poor filler integration. Another debated but commonly recommended practice is aspirating before injection. Although it does not guarantee that the needle is not inside a blood vessel, it may help reduce the risk of intravascular placement. Additionally, using the correct injection depth is crucial. Superficial injections tend to be safer, whereas deeper injections require greater caution to avoid vascular structures. Depositing excessive amounts of filler in one area should also be avoided, as large boluses can lead to compression of blood vessels, increasing the risk of ischemia. Lastly, choosing the appropriate filler for the specific indication is fundamental. High-viscosity fillers may have a greater potential for occlusion if injected intravascularly, whereas softer fillers tend to integrate more naturally into tissues.

5.2.2 Vascular anatomy and high-risk zones

A thorough understanding of lip vascular anatomy is vital for avoiding serious complications such as vascular occlusion or necrosis. The primary blood supply to the lips comes from the superior and inferior labial arteries, which are branches of the facial artery and run parallel to the vermilion border. Another high-risk vessel is the angular artery, which supplies the nasolabial fold and has the potential for embolization if filler is inadvertently injected into it. Additionally, the subdermal plexus contains numerous small vessels that can be compressed if excessive filler is injected in a concentrated area.

Certain areas of the lips and perioral region carry a higher risk of vascular compromise. The philtrum and Cupid's bow are particularly sensitive, as they are close to the superior labial artery. The nasolabial folds are another high-risk zone due to the presence of the angular artery, making filler injections in this area potentially hazardous. Deep perioral injections should also be performed cautiously to prevent compression of blood vessels supplying the lips. To reduce vascular risks, practitioners should always inject in small aliquots rather than large boluses, proceed slowly while observing for signs of vascular compromise, and consider using a blunt-tip cannula instead of a needle in high-risk areas to enhance safety.

5.3 Treatment of minor complications

Although minor complications are common, they can usually be managed effectively with conservative treatment. Recognizing and addressing these issues promptly can improve patient comfort and satisfaction.

5.3.1 Swelling and edema management

Swelling and edema are natural responses to filler injections, particularly since hyaluronic acid is highly hydrophilic and can draw water into the treated area. While mild swelling is expected, excessive inflammation can be uncomfortable for the patient. To manage this, cold compresses can be applied in the first 24 hours to reduce swelling. Keeping the head elevated while sleeping can also help minimize fluid accumulation in the lips. In cases of pronounced swelling, antihistamines may be useful, particularly if there is a mild allergic component. Patients should also be advised to limit excessive lip movement immediately after the procedure, as this can contribute to irritation and swelling.

5.3.2 Bruising and hematomas

Bruising occurs when small capillaries are disrupted during the injection process. While bruising is typically harmless, it can be esthetically concerning for the patient. Several measures can help reduce bruising, including the use of Arnica montana or bromelain supplements, which may speed up the resolution of bruises. Topical treatments containing vitamin K or arnica gel can also be beneficial. Gentle massage in cases of mild hematoma formation can help disperse the trapped blood and accelerate healing.

5.4 Corticosteroids for inflammatory reactions

In some cases, patients may develop excessive inflammation or hypersensitivity reactions following lip filler injections. When this occurs, low-dose *oral corticosteroids*, such as *prednisone* (5–10 mg for 3 days), can help control inflammation. For mild cases, *topical corticosteroids* may be sufficient. However, intralesional corticosteroid injections should be used with caution, as they can cause localized tissue atrophy if administered improperly.

5.5 Management of vascular complications

Vascular occlusion is one of the most serious complications of lip filler procedures. If left untreated, it can lead to *ischemia and tissue necrosis*, resulting in permanent damage. Prompt recognition and immediate intervention are critical to preventing severe outcomes.

5.5.1 Identifying vascular occlusion early

Key warning signs of vascular occlusion include blanching or whitening of the skin, intense pain beyond normal post-procedure discomfort, delayed capillary refill (>3 seconds) when applying pressure, and dusky or purple discoloration, indicating ischemia. If any of these signs occur, immediate action must be taken.

The first step is to stop injecting immediately. Massaging the area gently can sometimes help improve circulation. Applying warm compresses may assist in vasodilation, and topical nitroglycerin can also be considered to enhance blood flow.

5.5.2 Use of hyaluronidase for filler dissolution

In cases of suspected vascular occlusion, *hyaluronidase* should be injected promptly to dissolve the filler. The recommended dose is 150–300 units, injected in a grid-like pattern over the affected area. This process may need to be repeated every hour as necessary. Patients should be closely monitored for allergic reactions to hyaluronidase, as some individuals may exhibit hypersensitivity.

5.6 Additional treatments for severe cases

If ischemia persists despite initial measures, further interventions may be necessary. Nitroglycerin paste (2%) can be applied topically to promote vasodilation. Anticoagulants, such as aspirin or heparin, may be used if an embolic event is suspected. In severe cases, hyperbaric oxygen therapy (HBOT) can help restore oxygenation to ischemic tissues and reduce the risk of necrosis. If necrosis develops, wound care and surgical intervention may be required.

5.6.1 Resolution of nodules and granulomas

Delayed complications such as nodules and granulomas can develop weeks or months after the filler injection.

Mild inflammatory nodules can often be treated with massage or hyaluronidase injections to break down residual filler. If nodules persist, intralesional corticosteroids (triamcinolone 2.5–10 mg/ml) may be required. In cases where biofilm infection is suspected, a course of antibiotics (e.g., doxycycline or macrolides) may be beneficial.

In severe cases, surgical excision may be the only option, and histological analysis should be performed if there is any uncertainty about the nature of the lesion.

6. Conclusions

Effective complication management in lip filler procedures relies on prevention, early detection, and appropriate treatment strategies. Safe injection techniques and an understanding of vascular anatomy are essential for reducing risks. The "4.3" is a "standardized," simple, intuitive, and most importantly, reproducible technique that can be used in most patients, of both sexes, to achieve natural-looking lips, reducing the volume of filler injected (the treatment involves the use of about 0.7 ml) and the number of injections the patient has to undergo. By remaining vigilant and well-prepared, practitioners can ensure safe, effective, and esthetically optimal lip filler treatments while minimizing risks for their patients.

Author details

Francesco Castellaneta[1] and Mariagiovanna Lombardi[2*]

1 I.R.C.C.S. "Giovanni Paolo II", Bari, BA, Italy

2 Department of Plastic and Reconstructive Surgery, University of Naples Federico II, Napoli, Italy

*Address all correspondence to: lmariagiovanna@gmail.com

References

[1] Lupo MP. Hyaluronic acid fillers in facial rejuvenation. Seminars in Cutaneous Medicine and Surgery. 2006;**25**(3):122-126. DOI: 10.1016/j.sder.2006.06.011

[2] Koziej M, Trybus M, Hołda M, Polak J, Wnuk J, Brzegowy P, et al. Anatomical map of the facial artery for facial reconstruction and aesthetic procedures. Aesthetic Surgery Journal. 2019;**39**(11):1151-1162. DOI: 10.1093/asj/sjz028

[3] Nguyen JD, Duong H. Anatomy, head and neck: Labial artery. In: StatPearls [Internet]. Treasure Island (FL): StatPearls Publishing; 2023. p. 2023

[4] Cotofana S, Pretterklieber B, Lucius R, Frank K, Haas M, Schenck TL, et al. Distribution pattern of the superior and inferior labial arteries: Impact for safe upper and lower lip augmentation procedures. Plastic and Reconstructive Surgery. 2017;**139**(5):1075-1082. DOI: 10.1097/PRS.0000000000003244

[5] Lee SH, Gil YC, Choi YJ, Tansatit T, Kim HJ, Hu KS. Topographic anatomy of the superior labial artery for dermal filler injection. Plastic and Reconstructive Surgery. 2015;**135**(2):445-450. DOI: 10.1097/PRS.0000000000000858

[6] Luthra A. Shaping lips with fillers. Journal of Cutaneous and Aesthetic Surgery. 2015;**8**(3):139-142. DOI: 10.4103/0974-2077.167269

[7] Carruthers J, Narurkar VA. Management of the lips and mouth corners. In: Carruthers J, Carruthers A, editors. Soft Tissue Augmentation. Philadelphia: Saunders; 2006. pp. 109-119

[8] Smith SR, Lin X, Shamban A. Small gel particle hyaluronic acid injection technique for lip augmentation. Journal of Drugs in Dermatology. 2013;**12**(7):764-769

[9] Kanchwala SK, Holloway L, Bucky LP. Reliable soft tissue augmentation: A clinical comparison of injectable soft-tissue fillers for facial-volume augmentation. Annals of Plastic Surgery. 2005;**55**(1):30-35; discussion 35. DOI: 10.1097/01.sap.0000168292.69753.73

[10] Scheuer JF 3rd, Sieber DA, Pezeshk RA, Gassman AA, Campbell CF, Rohrich RJ. Facial danger zones: Techniques to maximize safety during soft-tissue filler injections. Plastic and Reconstructive Surgery. 2017;**139**(5):1103-1108. DOI: 10.1097/PRS.0000000000003309

[11] Castellaneta F, Lombardi M, D'Antonio S, Fabrizio T. The "4.3," a new filler lips technique. Journal of Cosmetic Dermatology. 2024;**24**(1):9-11. DOI: 10.1111/jocd.16601

Chapter 10

Exosome as a Therapeutic Agent in Cosmetic Dermatology

Gökçe Işıl Kurmuş and Selda Pelin Kartal

Abstract

Exosomes, nanosized extracellular vesicles, have emerged as crucial mediators of intercellular communication, facilitating the transfer of bioactive molecules such as proteins, lipids, and nucleic acids. In recent years, their potential application in cosmetic dermatology has attracted significant interest due to their ability to influence various biological processes, including skin regeneration, collagen synthesis, and the modulation of inflammation and oxidative stress. Exosomes derived from mesenchymal stem cells and other cell types have effectively promoted skin rejuvenation, reduced wrinkles, improved elasticity, and enhanced wound healing. Their use as a non-invasive, cell-free therapy offers distinct advantages, such as targeted delivery, minimal side effects, and improved bioavailability of therapeutic agents. Additionally, exosome-based formulations have shown promise in addressing photo-aging, pigmentation disorders, and hair loss. Despite these advancements, challenges remain regarding the standardization of exosome isolation, characterization, and large-scale clinical validation. This chapter aims to provide a comprehensive overview of the current and potential cosmetic applications of exosomes, emphasizing their role as innovative therapeutic agents capable of transforming cosmetic dermatology.

Keywords: exosome, cosmetic dermatology, skin regeneration, pigmentation disorders, esthetic medicine, hair loss

1. Introduction

Exosomes, a class of nanoscale extracellular vesicles, have attracted significant attention in biomedical research due to their crucial role in intercellular communication [1, 2]. These vesicles, typically 30–150 nm in diameter, are produced within the endosomal compartment of eukaryotic cells and serve as vehicles for transferring bioactive molecules, including proteins, lipids, nucleic acids, and metabolites [3, 4]. Exosomes have been identified in various biological fluids, such as amniotic fluid, cerebrospinal fluid, serum, and breast milk, underscoring their widespread presence and physiological significance [5–7].

Initially considered cellular debris, exosomes are recognized as fundamental mediators of numerous biological processes, including immune modulation, angiogenesis, tissue regeneration, and metabolic regulation [8–11]. Their ability to encapsulate molecular cargo within a lipid double-layer provides a protective environment that enhances the stability and functionality of their contents [1–4, 12]. This feature enables exosomes to facilitate targeted delivery of bioactive molecules to recipient cells through receptor-mediated endocytosis, direct membrane fusion, or micropinocytosis, thereby influencing cellular behavior and homeostasis [1, 6, 13].

Recent studies have highlighted the potential therapeutic applications of exosomes in various medical fields [10–14]. In oncology, exosomes have been explored as biomarkers for cancer diagnosis, prognosis, and vehicles for targeted drug delivery owing to their biocompatibility and low immunogenicity [15, 16]. Furthermore, exosome-based therapies have demonstrated promising results in regenerative medicine, particularly in treating cardiovascular diseases, neurodegenerative disorders, and immune-mediated conditions [7, 12, 15]. In dermatology, exosomes derived from mesenchymal stem cells (MSCs) have shown the ability to enhance skin repair, reduce inflammation, and modulate oxidative stress, making them a promising avenue for esthetic and therapeutic interventions [3–7].

The skin, as the human body's largest organ, serves as a protective barrier against environmental stressors while maintaining homeostasis through a complex interplay of cellular and molecular mechanisms [4–7]. Various factors, including aging, UV radiation, pollution, and genetic predisposition, contribute to skin deterioration, leading to wrinkling, pigmentation disorders, hair loss, and impaired wound healing [2–5]. There is an increasing demand for innovative, non-invasive therapeutic modalities that address skin-related concerns at a cellular level [3–5].

In this chapter, we explore the emerging role of exosomes in cosmetic dermatology, focusing on their potential applications in skin rejuvenation and anti-aging, wound healing, and scar treatment, pigmentation disorders such as melasma and hyperpigmentation, and hair loss treatment, including alopecia. By exploring the mechanisms underlying exosome-mediated skin regeneration and repair, we aim to provide a comprehensive overview of their therapeutic potential, current challenges, and future directions in cosmetic dermatology.

2. Biogenesis and mechanisms of action of exosomes

Exosomes originate from the endosomal system through a well-coordinated biogenesis process involving multiple cellular pathways [1–3]. Their formation begins with the invagination of the plasma membrane to create early endosomes, which subsequently mature into late endosomes or multivesicular bodies (MVBs) containing intraluminal vesicles (ILVs) [13, 17]. Upon fusion of MVBs with the plasma membrane, ILVs are secreted into the extracellular space as exosomes, facilitating intercellular communication by transferring biomolecular cargo such as proteins, lipids, and nucleic acids [13, 17].

The Endosomal Sorting Complex Required for Transport (ESCRT) plays a central role in exosome biogenesis [13, 17]. ESCRT-dependent mechanisms involve a sequential recruitment of ESCRT-0, -I, -II, and -III, which facilitate cargo selection and membrane cleavage [13]. However, alternative pathways, such as the tetraspanin- and lipid raft-mediated mechanisms, also contribute to ILV formation and exosome secretion, indicating a degree of overlap and complexity in exosome biogenesis [13]. Rab GTPases, including Rab27, Rab11, and Rab35, regulate exosome trafficking and secretion by modulating MVB transport and attachment at the plasma membrane [13].

Once released, exosomes interact with recipient cells through various uptake mechanisms, including direct membrane fusion, receptor-mediated endocytosis, clathrin- and caveolin-dependent internalization, and micropinocytosis [13, 17]. The uptake process is often influenced by exosome surface molecules, such as integrins, tetraspanins (CD9, CD63, and CD81), and adhesion proteins, mediating targeted interactions with recipient cells [13]. Cholesterol- and sphingolipid-rich domains enhance exosomal stability and facilitate their fusion with recipient cell membranes [13].

Functionally, exosomes participate in diverse physiological and pathological processes. In skin biology, exosomes derived from mesenchymal stem cells (MSCs) modulate wound healing by enhancing fibroblast proliferation, extracellular matrix remodeling, and angiogenesis [18]. Studies have demonstrated that MSC-derived exosomes promote collagen synthesis and keratinocyte migration by activating the TGF-β and Wnt/β-catenin signaling pathways [18]. Additionally, MSC exosomes regulate inflammatory responses by suppressing pro-inflammatory cytokines and enhancing anti-inflammatory mediators, a mechanism relevant to chronic inflammatory dermatoses such as psoriasis and atopic dermatitis [4, 18].

The therapeutic potential of exosomes extends beyond skin repair to include applications in regenerative medicine, oncology, and neurodegenerative disorders [15]. For instance, exosomes have been shown to reduce UV-induced skin aging by reducing oxidative stress and promoting dermal fibroblast proliferation [3]. In cosmetic dermatology, exosomes have shown promise in addressing pigmentation disorders such as melasma and post-inflammatory hyperpigmentation by regulating melanogenesis [6]. Studies indicate that exosomes derived from MSCs can inhibit melanin synthesis by downregulating tyrosinase activity and reducing melanocyte oxidative stress [5]. Additionally, exosomal microRNAs play a regulatory role in melanogenesis by modulating the expression of tyrosinase, influencing melanocyte-inducing transcription factor-dependent signaling pathways, and directly affecting melanin production, thereby altering pigmentation homeostasis [14].

Despite their promise, challenges remain in standardizing exosome isolation, characterization, and therapeutic application. Current isolation techniques, including ultracentrifugation, immunoaffinity capture, and microfluidic separation, vary in output and purity, necessitating further optimization for clinical translation [17]. Additionally, ensuring the expandability and safety of exosome-based therapies requires thorough regulatory evaluation and reproducibility in clinical studies [5, 8].

As research advances, a deeper understanding of exosome biogenesis and mechanisms of action will enable the development of novel therapeutic strategies for dermatological and systemic diseases. Continued investigation into exosomal cargo selection, targeted delivery, and functional modifications will further enhance their applicability in precision medicine and regenerative therapies.

3. Exosomes in cosmetic dermatology: Current applications

3.1 Skin rejuvenation and anti-aging

Aging is a complex biological process influenced by intrinsic and extrinsic factors, leading to structural and functional changes in the skin [2]. Exosomes have emerged as promising therapeutic agents in anti-aging treatments due to their role in cellular communication, extracellular matrix (ECM) remodeling, and oxidative stress reduction [9, 16]. Their ability to transfer bioactive molecules, including microRNAs, proteins, and lipids, makes them potent modulators of fibroblast activity and collagen homeostasis [6–8].

Multiple preclinical studies have demonstrated the efficacy of exosome-based therapies in skin rejuvenation. Oh et al. reported that human-induced pluripotent stem cell-derived exosomes reversed UV-induced photoaging by reducing the expression of senescence markers, such as β-galactosidase, and increasing collagen type I production [19]. Similarly, Liang et al. found that subcutaneous injection of adipose-derived stem cell exosomes increases dermal thickness, restores the balance of type I and III collagen, and reduces matrix metalloproteinase expression, leading to improved skin structure and delayed aging-related changes in photoaged rat skin [20].

Clinical studies further support the application of exosomes in esthetic dermatology. A 12-week prospective, randomized, split-face study by Park et al. evaluated the efficacy of adipose tissue stem cell-derived exosomes combined with microneedling for skin rejuvenation. The study demonstrated significant improvements in skin hydration, elasticity, and wrinkle reduction compared to placebo-treated areas [21]. Proffer et al. conducted a prospective, single-arm, non-randomized longitudinal study to evaluate the safety and efficacy of topical platelet-derived exosomes for skin rejuvenation. In this clinical trial, the topical application of platelet-derived exosomes significantly improved skin health parameters, including erythema, pigmentation, luminosity, and wrinkle reduction, within 6 weeks. The treatment was well-tolerated, with no significant adverse effects and high participant satisfaction [22]. Chernoff et al. conducted a clinical study to evaluate the effects of combining topical dermal infusion of exosomes with injected calcium hydroxylapatite (CaHA) for enhanced tissue biostimulation. The study involved 40 patients, who were divided into different groups receiving either topical exosome treatment alone, CaHA injections alone, or a combination of both. The study demonstrated that both treatments individually improved skin tone, texture, and vascularity, while their combination led to faster and more pronounced rejuvenation effects [23]. In a clinical trial, Jo et al. investigated the effects of *Lactobacillus plantarum*-derived extracellular vesicles (LpEVs) on skin aging. Their findings demonstrated that topical application of LpEVs for 4 weeks significantly reduced eye wrinkles, improved skin elasticity, enhanced hydration, and increased dermal density in 16 volunteers [24].

Despite their promising clinical outcomes, the widespread adoption of exosome-based therapies in skin rejuvenation faces challenges related to standardization, including variability in isolation techniques, purity, and bioactivity. Additionally, long-term safety and regulatory considerations remain critical factors requiring further investigation. However, advancements in exosome engineering, optimized delivery systems, and controlled clinical studies hold the potential to refine their therapeutic applications. By overcoming these limitations, exosome-based treatments could establish a new standard in esthetic dermatology, offering safe, effective, and reproducible solutions for skin aging and rejuvenation.

3.2 Wound healing and scar treatment

Wound healing is a highly coordinated biological process involving inflammation, cell proliferation, extracellular matrix (ECM) remodeling, and tissue regeneration [1]. Various intrinsic and extrinsic factors, including age, oxidative stress, and immune dysfunction, can impair this process, leading to delayed wound closure or pathological scarring [16]. Exosomes have emerged as a promising therapeutic modality in wound healing due to their ability to mediate intercellular communication, modulate immune responses, and promote angiogenesis [2, 11]. Their regenerative potential is primarily attributed to their bioactive cargo, including growth factors, microRNAs (miRNAs), and extracellular vesicle-associated proteins, which facilitate cellular proliferation, migration, and tissue remodeling [11].

Several studies have demonstrated the effectiveness of exosomes in enhancing wound repair. Wang et al. demonstrate that exosomes derived from human adipose mesenchymal stem cells (ASC-Exos) promote scarless wound healing in a murine model. ASC-Exos increases the collagen III/collagen I and TGF-β3/TGF-β1 ratios while preventing fibroblast differentiation into myofibroblasts, thereby reducing scar formation [25]. In another study, Zhang et al. indicate that exosomes derived from human-induced pluripotent stem cell-derived mesenchymal stem cells (hiPSC-MSC-Exos) significantly enhance cutaneous wound healing. The results demonstrate that hiPSC-MSC-Exos promotes re-epithelialization, reduces scar width, and increases collagen synthesis. Additionally, these exosomes facilitate angiogenesis by stimulating the formation and maturation of new blood vessels [26].

Beyond wound closure, exosomes play a critical role in scar remodeling. Excessive fibroblast activation and disorganized collagen deposition often lead to hypertrophic scars or keloids, which pose significant esthetic and functional concerns. Keloids are characterized by excessive fibroblast proliferation and abnormal ECM deposition [27]. Recent studies suggest that exosomes may regulate keloid formation by targeting fibrotic pathways [5, 27].

Exosomes regulate keloid and hypertrophic scar formation by inhibiting fibroblast proliferation and promoting apoptosis. Modulating the TGF-β/Smad signaling pathway suppresses collagen synthesis while reducing inflammation and angiogenesis [4, 27]. These mechanisms position exosomes as promising therapeutic agents for managing pathological scarring [4, 27].

Clinical applications of exosomes in wound healing and scar treatment are gaining traction. A 12-week, prospective, double-blind, randomized, split-face clinical trial included 25 patients who underwent three consecutive fractional CO_2 laser sessions, with one side of the face treated with adipose tissue stem cell-derived exosomes and the other with a control gel [28]. The study demonstrated that exosome-treated areas showed more significant improvement, shorter recovery time, and fewer side effects than control-treated areas. These findings suggest that exosomes may enhance the therapeutic outcomes of laser resurfacing for atrophic acne scars [28].

Despite the promising findings, several challenges remain regarding the clinical translation of exosome-based therapies. Exosome isolation, purification, and dosage standardization remain crucial challenges in ensuring consistency and reproducibility across studies. Additionally, regulatory frameworks for the therapeutic application of exosomes in wound healing and scar treatment require further refinement to address safety concerns and optimize therapeutic efficacy.

3.3 Pigmentation disorders

Pigmentation disorders, including melasma and post-inflammatory hyperpigmentation (PIH), result from dysregulated melanogenesis, excessive melanosome transfer, and chronic inflammation [5]. Factors such as ultraviolet (UV) exposure, hormonal changes, and oxidative stress contribute to their pathogenesis [9]. Exosomes have emerged as promising therapeutic agents due to their ability to modulate melanocyte activity, melanin synthesis, and inflammatory responses [5, 9].

Exosomes derived from mesenchymal stem cells (MSC-exos) and adipose-derived stem cells (ADSC-exos) have been shown to regulate pigmentation by modulating melanin-related signaling pathways [5, 9]. They also play a role in PIH by modulating inflammatory responses [5]. A study by Cicero et al. revealed that keratinocyte-derived exosomes enhance melanogenesis by increasing melanosomal protein expression and activity in melanocytes, with their effects further amplified by UVB exposure [29]. Kim et al. identified an alternative interaction between human umbilical cord blood-derived mesenchymal stem cell (hUCB-MSC) exosomes and melanocytes, demonstrating that these exosomes inhibited melanin synthesis by regulating microphthalmia-associated transcription factor (MITF) through activation of the extracellular signal-regulated kinase (ERK) pathway [30].

A prospective, split-face, double-blind, randomized, placebo-controlled clinical study evaluated the skin-brightening efficacy of adipose tissue-derived stem cell exosomes in 21 female participants with hyperpigmentation [31]. The results demonstrated that the exosome-containing formulation significantly reduced melanin levels compared to placebo, with effects observed after 4 weeks of treatment. However, the melanin-reduction effect diminished over time, highlighting the need for improved transdermal delivery methods to enhance clinical efficacy [31].

Despite promising results, challenges remain in standardizing exosome isolation, dosing, and clinical application, highlighting the need for large-scale, multicenter trials to confirm long-term efficacy and safety. Regulatory approval of exosome-based depigmentation therapies is also in its early stages, with ongoing investigations into biocompatibility and long-term pigmentation modulation. However, exosome-based therapies provide a non-invasive, cell-free alternative to traditional depigmentation treatments, reducing side effects associated with hydroquinone and corticosteroids and leading the way for next-generation precision medicine in dermatology.

3.4 Hair loss treatment

Hair loss, particularly androgenetic alopecia (AGA) and alopecia areata (AA), is a prevalent condition with significant psychosocial impacts [32]. Conventional treatments, including minoxidil, finasteride, and platelet-rich plasma therapy, provide varying degrees of efficacy but often fail to achieve sustained hair regrowth [33]. Recent research has highlighted the therapeutic potential of exosome-based therapies in hair follicle (HF) regeneration due to their role in cellular communication, extracellular matrix remodeling, and modulation of inflammatory and growth factor signaling pathways [32, 33].

Exosomes derived from adipose-derived stem cells (ADSC-Exos) have demonstrated efficacy in promoting hair follicle regeneration by stimulating dermal papilla cells (DPCs) and activating Wnt/β-catenin signaling [33]. Hu et al. found that ADSC-Exos significantly increased hair follicle density, dermal thickness, and anagen phase duration in a murine model of AGA. The study revealed that exosomal microRNAs (miRNAs), particularly miR-218-5p, enhanced HF proliferation by downregulating SFRP2, an inhibitor of β-catenin signaling [34]. Another study reported that ADSC-Exos reversed DHT-induced suppression of DPC proliferation through SMAD3 pathway inhibition, leading to increased β-catenin activity and HF stem cell renewal [35]. Exosomes derived from dermal papilla cells (DPC-Exos) have also shown regenerative effects in HF cycling. Kwack et al. demonstrated that DPC-Exos upregulated the secretion of growth factors such as hepatocyte growth factor (HGF), insulin-like growth factor-1 (IGF-1), and keratinocyte growth factor (KGF), leading to prolonged anagen phase and delayed catagen onset in human HF organoid models [36].

Beyond preclinical studies, clinical evidence supports the potential of exosome-based therapies for hair loss treatment. A randomized, double-blind, vehicle-controlled clinical trial evaluated the efficacy and safety of adipose-derived stem cell constituent extract (ADSC-CE) for hair regeneration in AGA [37]. The study found that adipose-derived stem cell constituent extract (ADSC-CE) significantly increased hair count and thickness in patients with androgenetic alopecia over 16 weeks, with noticeable effects beginning at week 8. A prospective study included 30 male patients aged 22–65 with Norwood-Hamilton type III-VI AGA, assessing the effects of foreskin-derived mesenchymal stromal cell exosome injections on hair density and patient satisfaction [38]. The results demonstrated a significant increase in hair density at the 4th and 12th weeks post-treatment, with sustained patient satisfaction.

Despite these promising findings, challenges remain in standardizing exosome-based hair loss treatments. Variability in exosome isolation methods, dosage, and delivery mechanisms necessitates further large-scale clinical trials to establish safety and efficacy. Moreover, regulatory approval remains a significant challenge, as no exosome-based product has yet received FDA approval for alopecia treatment. As research progresses, future studies focusing on long-term efficacy, safety, and optimal treatment protocols will be crucial for integrating exosome-based therapies into mainstream dermatological practice.

4. Challenges and future perspectives

Despite the growing interest in exosome-based therapies for cosmetic dermatology, several challenges must be addressed before their widespread clinical use. One of the main challenges is the lack of standardized methods for exosome isolation, purification, and production [4]. Current techniques, such as ultracentrifugation and size-exclusion chromatography, often lead to variability in exosome quality, concentration, and bioactivity, making it challenging to ensure reproducibility in clinical applications and limiting the scalability of production for commercial use [39]. Additionally, the stability of exosome formulations remains a concern, as they are sensitive to storage conditions, requiring advancements in preservation techniques to maintain their therapeutic potential.

Regulatory challenges also pose significant barriers to exosome-based treatments. Exosomes have no universal classification, as they can be considered biologics, cell-free therapies, or drug delivery systems, depending on their source and intended application. Different regulatory agencies impose varying requirements for safety and efficacy assessments, slowing the approval process and clinical adoption of exosome-based dermatological treatments [40]. To overcome this, comprehensive clinical trials are needed to establish their long-term safety, effectiveness, and optimal usage in cosmetic procedures.

Other important considerations are patient safety and ethical concerns. Since exosomes can be derived from multiple sources, including stem cells and blood products, issues related to donor consent, potential immune reactions, and contamination risks must be carefully managed [41]. While autologous exosome therapies may reduce immunogenic risks, they are time-consuming and expensive, making allogeneic sources more practical for commercial use [42]. However, the safety of allogeneic exosomes requires further study to ensure they do not trigger unwanted immune responses or transfer unintended biological material [42].

Looking ahead, genetically engineered exosomes present exciting possibilities for improving their therapeutic effects. By modifying exosomes to carry specific bioactive molecules, researchers aim to enhance their ability to stimulate collagen production, regulate pigmentation, and promote hair growth. Additionally, advanced delivery systems, such as microneedle patches, hydrogel carriers, and nanotechnology-based formulations, are being explored to improve the absorption and efficacy of exosome treatments in dermatology [7–14]. These innovations could lead to more targeted and long-lasting results, making exosome-based therapies more accessible and effective.

5. Conclusions

Exosome-based therapies represent a promising advancement in cosmetic dermatology, offering cell-free solutions for skin rejuvenation, scar treatment, pigmentation disorders, and hair loss. Their ability to enhance cellular communication, tissue repair, and regenerative processes has positioned them as a potential alternative to traditional treatments. However, standardization, regulatory approval, and long-term safety challenges must be addressed before exosome-based products can become widely available.

Future research should optimize exosome production, refine delivery methods, and conduct large-scale clinical trials to validate their safety and effectiveness. Collaboration between scientists, clinicians, and regulatory bodies will be essential to establish guidelines that ensure the responsible development of exosome therapies. With continued progress, exosome-based treatments have the potential to redefine cosmetic dermatology, providing innovative, non-invasive solutions for skin and hair concerns.

Author details

Gökçe Işıl Kurmuş* and Selda Pelin Kartal
Department of Dermatology and Venereology, Ankara Etlik City Hospital, Ankara, Turkey

*Address all correspondence to: isilkurmus@gmail.com

References

[1] De A, Chakraborty D, Agarwal I, Sarda A. Present and future use of exosomes in dermatology. Indian Journal of Dermatology. 2024;**69**:461-470. DOI: 10.4103/ijd.ijd_491_23

[2] Olumesi KR, Goldberg DJ. A review of exosomes and their application in cutaneous medical aesthetics. Journal of Cosmetic Dermatology. 2023;**22**:2628-2634. DOI: 10.1111/jocd.15930

[3] Bai G, Truong TM, Pathak GN, Benoit L, Rao B. Clinical applications of exosomes in cosmetic dermatology. Skin Health and Disease. 2024;**4**:e348. DOI: 10.1002/ski2.348

[4] Yu H, Feng H, Zeng H, Wu Y, Zhang Q, Yu J, et al. Exosomes: The emerging mechanisms and potential clinical applications in dermatology. International Journal of Biological Sciences. 2024;**20**:1778-1795. DOI: 10.7150/ijbs.92897

[5] Villarreal-Gómez LJ, Origel-Lucio S, Hernández-Hernández DA, Pérez-González GL. Use of exosomes for cosmetics applications. Cosmetics. 2025;**12**:9

[6] Schur N, Samman L, Shah M, Dukharan V, Stegura C, Broughton L, et al. Exosomes: Historical evolution and emerging roles in dermatology. Journal of Cosmetic Dermatology. 2025;**24**:e16769. DOI: 10.1111/jocd.16769

[7] Miller J, Chen G, Hayag MV. A review of exosomes in regenerative cosmetic dermatology. Molecular Frontiers Journal. 2023;**7**:64-70

[8] Novis T, Menezes AHG, Lima LCV, Lötvall J, do Nascimento IJB, Takiya CM. The therapeutic, diagnostic, and prognostic values of extracellular vesicles (exosomes) in dermatology: A systematic review. JAAD Reviews. 2024;**1**:135-174. DOI: 10.1016/j.jdrv.2024.06.006

[9] Shah M, Dukharan V, Broughton L, Stegura C, Schur N, Samman L, et al. Exosomes for aesthetic dermatology: A comprehensive literature review and update. Journal of Cosmetic Dermatology. 2025;**24**:e16766. DOI: 10.1111/jocd.16766

[10] Thakur A, Shah D, Rai D, Parra DC, Pathikonda S, Kurilova S, et al. Therapeutic values of exosomes in cosmetics, skin care, tissue regeneration, and dermatological diseases. Cosmetics. 2023;**10**:65

[11] Dal'Forno-Dini T, Birck MS, Rocha M, Bagatin E. Exploring the reality of exosomes in dermatology. Anais Brasileiros de Dermatologia. 2025;**100**:121-130. DOI: 10.1016/j.abd.2024.09.002

[12] Yousefian F, Espinoza L, Yadlapati S, Lorenc ZP, Gold M. A comprehensive review of the medical and cosmetic applications of exosomes in dermatology. Journal of Cosmetic Dermatology. 2024;**23**:1224-1228. DOI: 10.1111/jocd.16149

[13] McBride JD, Rodriguez-Menocal L, Badiavas EV. Extracellular vesicles as biomarkers and therapeutics in dermatology: A focus on exosomes. The Journal of Investigative Dermatology. 2017;**137**:1622-1629

[14] Xiong M, Zhang Q, Hu W, Zhao C, Lv W, Yi Y, et al. The novel mechanisms and applications of exosomes in dermatology and cutaneous medical aesthetics. Pharmacological Research. 2021;**166**:105490. DOI: 10.1016/j.phrs.2021.105490

[15] Szwedowicz U, Łapińska Z, Gajewska-Naryniecka A, Choromańska A. Exosomes and other extracellular vesicles with high therapeutic potential: Their applications in oncology, neurology, and dermatology. Molecules. 2022;**27**:1303. DOI: 10.3390/molecules27041303

[16] McGraw IT, Wilson EE, Behfar A, Paradise CR, Rohrich RJ, Wyles SP. Evolving role of exosomes in plastic and reconstructive surgery and dermatology. Plastic and Reconstructive Surgery. Global Open. 2024;**12**:e6061. DOI: 10.1097/GOX.0000000000006061

[17] Chen J, Li P, Zhang T, Xu Z, Huang X, Wang R, et al. Review on strategies and Technologies for Exosome Isolation and Purification. Frontiers in Bioengineering and Biotechnology. 2022;**9**:811971. DOI: 10.3389/fbioe.2021.811971

[18] Quiñones-Vico MI, Sanabria-de la Torre R, Sánchez-Díaz M, Sierra-Sánchez Á, Montero-Vílchez T, Fernández-González A, et al. The role of exosomes derived from mesenchymal stromal cells in dermatology. Frontiers in Cell and Development Biology. 2021;**9**:647012. DOI: 10.3389/fcell.2021.647012

[19] Oh M, Lee J, Kim YJ, Rhee WJ, Park JH. Exosomes derived from human induced pluripotent stem cells ameliorate the aging of skin fibroblasts. International Journal of Molecular Sciences. 2018;**19**(6):1715. DOI: 10.3390/ijms19061715

[20] Liang JX, Liao X, Li SH, Jiang X, Li ZH, Wu YD, et al. Antiaging properties of exosomes from adipose-derived mesenchymal stem cells in Photoaged rat skin. BioMed Research International. 2020;**21**(2020):6406395. DOI: 10.1155/2020/6406395

[21] Park GH, Kwon HH, Seok J, Yang SH, Lee J, Park BC, et al. Efficacy of combined treatment with human adipose tissue stem cell-derived exosome-containing solution and microneedling for facial skin aging: A 12-week prospective, randomized, split-face study. Journal of Cosmetic Dermatology. 2023;**22**:3418-3426. DOI: 10.1111/jocd.15872

[22] Proffer SL, Paradise CR, DeGrazia E, Halaas Y, Durairaj KK, Somenek M, et al. Efficacy and tolerability of topical platelet exosomes for skin rejuvenation: Six-week results. Aesthetic Surgery Journal. 2022;**42**:1185-1193. DOI: 10.1093/asj/sjac149

[23] Chernoff G. Combining topical dermal infused exosomes with injected calcium hydroxylapatite for enhanced tissue biostimulation. Journal of Cosmetic Dermatology. 2023;**22**(Suppl. 1):15-27. DOI: 10.1111/jocd.15695

[24] Jo CS, Myung CH, Yoon YC, Ahn BH, Min JW, Seo WS, et al. The effect of lactobacillus plantarum extracellular vesicles from Korean women in their 20s on skin aging. Current Issues in Molecular Biology. 2022;**44**:526-540. DOI: 10.3390/cimb44020036

[25] Wang L, Hu L, Zhou X, Xiong Z, Zhang C, Shehada HMA, et al. Exosomes secreted by human adipose mesenchymal stem cells promote scarless cutaneous repair by regulating extracellular matrix remodelling. Scientific Reports. 2017;7:13321. DOI: 10.1038/s41598-017-12919-x

[26] Zhang J, Guan J, Niu X, Hu G, Guo S, Li Q, et al. Exosomes released from human induced pluripotent stem cells-derived MSCs facilitate cutaneous wound healing by promoting collagen synthesis and angiogenesis. Journal of

Translational Medicine. 2015;**13**:49. DOI: 10.1186/s12967-015-0417-0

[27] Zhong Y, Zhang Y, Yu A, Zhang Z, Deng Z, Xiong K, et al. Therapeutic role of exosomes and conditioned medium in keloid and hypertrophic scar and possible mechanisms. Frontiers in Physiology. 2023;**14**:1247734

[28] Kwon HH, Yang SH, Lee J, Park BC, Park KY, Jung JY, et al. Combination treatment with human adipose tissue stem cell-derived exosomes and fractional CO2 laser for acne scars: A 12-week prospective, double-blind, randomized,split-face study. Acta Dermato-Venereologica. 2020;**100**(18):adv00310. DOI: 10.2340/00015555-3666

[29] Cicero A, Delevoye C, Gilles-Marsens F, Loew D, Dingli F, Guéré C, et al. Exosomes released by keratinocytes modulate melanocyte pigmentation. Nature Communications. 2015;**6**:7506. DOI: 10.1038/ncomms8506

[30] Kim ES, Jeon HB, Lim H, Shin JH, Park SJ, Jo YK, et al. Conditioned media from human umbilical cord blood-derived mesenchymal stem cells inhibits Melanogenesis by promoting proteasomal degradation of MITF. PLoS One. 2015;**10**:e0128078. DOI: 10.1371/journal.pone.0128078

[31] Cho BS, Lee J, Won Y, Duncan DI, Jin RC, Lee J, et al. Skin brightening efficacy of exosomes derived from human adipose tissue-derived stem/stromal cells: A prospective, Split-face, Randomized Placebo-Controlled Study. Cosmetics. 2020;**7**:90. DOI: 10.3390/cosmetics7040090

[32] Gupta AK, Wang T, Rapaport JA. Systematic review of exosome treatment in hair restoration: Preliminary evidence, safety, and future directions. Journal of Cosmetic Dermatology. 2023;**22**:2424-2433. DOI: 10.1111/jocd.15869

[33] Cheng M, Ma C, Chen HD, Wu Y, Xu XG. The roles of exosomes in regulating hair follicle growth. Clinical, Cosmetic and Investigational Dermatology. 2024;**17**:1603-1612. DOI: 10.2147/CCID.S465963

[34] Hu S, Li Z, Lutz H, Huang K, Su T, Cores J, et al. Dermal exosomes containing miR-218-5p promote hair regeneration by regulating β-catenin signaling. Science Advances. 2020;**6**:eaba1685

[35] Liang Y, Tang X, Zhang X, Cao C, Yu M, Wan M. Adipose mesenchymal stromal cell-derived exosomes carrying MiR-122-5p antagonize the inhibitory effect of dihydrotestosterone on hair follicles by targeting the TGF-β1/SMAD3 Signaling pathway. International Journal of Molecular Sciences. 2023;**24**:5703. DOI: 10.3390/ijms24065703

[36] Kwack MH, Seo CH, Gangadaran P, Ahn BC, Kim MK, Kim JC, et al. Exosomes derived from human dermal papilla cells promote hair growth in cultured human hair follicles and augment the hair-inductive capacity of cultured dermal papilla spheres. Experimental Dermatology. 2019;**28**:854-857. DOI: 10.1111/exd.13927

[37] Tak YJ, Lee SY, Cho AR, Kim YS. A randomized, double-blind, vehicle-controlled clinical study of hair regeneration using adipose-derived stem cell constituent extract in androgenetic alopecia. Stem Cells Translational Medicine. 2020;**9**:839-849. DOI: 10.1002/sctm.19-0410

[38] Ersan M, Ozer E, Akin O, Tasli PN, Sahin F. Effectiveness of exosome treatment in androgenetic alopecia: Outcomes of a prospective study.

Aesthetic Plastic Surgery. 2024;**48**:4262-4271. DOI: 10.1007/s00266-024-04332-3

[39] Liu WZ, Ma ZJ, Kang XW. Current status and outlook of advances in exosome isolation. Analytical and Bioanalytical Chemistry. 2022;**414**:7123-7141. DOI: 10.1007/s00216-022-04253-7

[40] Rodriguez C, Porcello A, Chemali M, Raffoul W, Marques C, Scaletta C, et al. Medicalized aesthetic uses of exosomes and cell culture-conditioned media: Opening an advanced care era for biologically inspired cutaneous Prejuvenation and rejuvenation. Cosmetics. 2024;**11**:154. DOI: 10.3390/cosmetics11050154

[41] Volarevic V, Markovic BS, Gazdic M, Volarevic A, Jovicic N, Arsenijevic N, et al. Ethical and safety issues of stem cell-based therapy. International Journal of Medical Sciences. 2018;**15**:36-45. DOI: 10.7150/ijms.21666

[42] Li C, Zhao H, Cheng L, Wang B. Allogeneic vs. autologous mesenchymal stem/stromal cells in their medication practice. Cell & Bioscience. 2021;**11**:187. DOI: 10.1186/s13578-021-00698-y